Ayurveda

FOR WOMEN

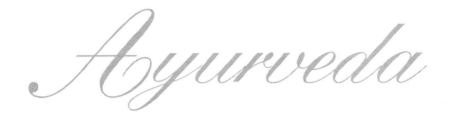

Ayurveda

FOR WOMEN

A Guide to
Vitality and Health

DR. ROBERT E. SVOBODA

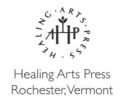

Healing Arts Press
Rochester, Vermont

Healing Arts Press
One Park Street
Rochester, Vermont 05767
www.InnerTraditions.com

Healing Arts Press is a division of Inner Traditions International

*Note to the reader: This book is intended as an informational guide. The remedies,
approaches, and techniques described herein are meant to supplement, and not to be a
substitute for, professional medical care or treatment. They should not be used to treat a
serious ailment without prior consultation with a qualified health care professional.*

Library of Congress Cataloging-in-Publication Data

Svoboda, Robert.
    Ayurveda for women : a guide to vitality and health / Robert E. Svoboda.
        p. cm.
    Previously published by David & Charles Publishers of the UK in 1999.
    Includes bibliographical references and index.
    ISBN 0-89281-939-1 (alk. paper)
        1. Women—Health and hygiene. 2. Medicine, Ayurvedic. I. Title.

    RA778 .S946 2000
    615.5'3'082—dc21

00-059784

Printed and bound in Canada

10 9 8 7 6 5 4 3 2

Text design and layout by Priscilla H. Baker
This book was typeset in Caslon and Gill Sans, with Kuenstler as a display face

Contents

Acknowledgments

Many people have assisted me in this book's development, including Judith Morrison and Dr. Will Foster, as well as the whole staff at David & Charles, enthusiastically led by Fiona Eaton and seconded by Ali Myer. A big "thank you" to all of you, and to Margaret Mahan, the person who deserves the greatest credit for conceiving the idea for this book and for working hard to get it out in its original form.

Introduction

Ayurveda is India's traditional system of health and healing. Perhaps humankind's most ancient medical system, it—or something similar—was already being practiced in India many thousands of years ago. Ayurveda explores life in all its layers and pays more attention to an organism's energies and their functions than to the structures which contain them. It concerns itself less with quantity of life than with life's quality, and with those qualities in our environments and ourselves that promote an individual's state of health or ill health on every level of existence.

Although Ayurveda takes all of embodied life (including animals and plants) as its field of activity, this book focuses on the female human being. It addresses feminine physical, mental, emotional, and spiritual realities, and the many areas of women's lives that are unique to them as women. We begin with Ayurveda's basics—principles that are as true for stallions and pear trees as they are for people!—and proceed to explore women's concerns in three sections that correspond to the three ages of a woman's life. Each of these introduces and explains those aspects of Ayurveda that are most relevant to that age. As a whole, the book seeks to deliver a faithful image of the reality that Ayurveda was created to mirror: the comedy and the drama, the trees and the forest—in short, everything that is suitable and unsuitable for promoting health and happiness in an individual human life.

Historical Origins

Ayurveda originated within the tradition of the *Vedas*, India's ancient books of wisdom, which were "discovered" by seers known as *rishis*, enlightened experimenters who worked within the "laboratories" of their own awarenesses. Out of the abundance of their compassion they systematized their findings for their less enlightened posterity, and anyone who is willing to cultivate a little interiority can stick her toe into this lake of knowledge.

The *Vedas* took on their current form at some point during the second millenium B.C., although this version is derived from much earlier versions which are now lost. Ayurveda developed from the youngest of the *Vedas*, the *Atharva Veda*. When, during the first millenium B.C., Indian culture entered its Golden Age, the first substantial texts of Ayurveda were codified: the *Charaka Samhita*, which deals mainly with internal medicine, and the *Sushruta Samhita*, which focuses on surgery. Ayurveda continued to flourish over the next few centuries, and new texts were continually being written. The Ayurvedic text used most widely today, the *Ashtanga Hridaya of Vagbhata*, was written around A.D. 700. It consists of a backbone formed by condensing the works of *Charaka* and *Sushruta*, fleshed out with newly described diseases and therapies.

During India's medieval period, political turmoil began to interfere with the development of Ayurveda, and what appeared at the time to be a death blow to the system was delivered in 1835 by Lord Macaulay. He directed that thenceforth European medical knowledge should be encouraged exclusively in all areas of India governed by the East India Company. Having thus lost all government approval and patronage, Ayurveda had to retreat underground, the flame of its traditions tended carefully as before by generations of dedicated adherents. But even during this period of persecution Ayurveda contributed generously to Western medicine. During the nineteenth century, the Germans translated from *Sushruta's* treatise details of an operation for the repair of damaged noses and ears. This operation, which now appears in modern textbooks as the pedicle graft, led to the development of plastic surgery as an independent specialization. *Sushruta* is today regarded by plastic surgeons the world over as the father of their craft.

With the assertion of Indian nationalism at the dawn of the twentieth century, interest in Indian art and science was reawakened and Ayurveda began a gradual revival, which continues today. This parallels the growing awareness in the West that there is more to life and health than physical existence alone.

A Note of Encouragement

Don't be concerned, as you read through this book, when you find yourself confronted by unfamiliar words or concepts. If you simply ignore them at the beginning, and work instead toward grasping the essence of what is written, you will find it easy later on to comprehend them when you meet them again. In this way the book itself will do most of the work of educating you, leaving you to turn your attention inward to the places where it is most needed.

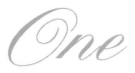

THE FOUNDATIONS
OF HEALTH

Although Ayurveda is renowned as a medical system, medicine is but a small portion of the voluminous tapestry of its knowledge. A well-tuned Ayurvedic physician will be versed in elements of cookery, music, dance, astrology, language, spirituality, and of several other of the disciplines that contribute to making a life well lived. I was fortunate to have had as an Ayurvedic mentor the Aghori Vimalananda, a genuine Renaissance man who lived Ayurveda's principles daily. His example showed me time and again how essential such supplementary knowledge is, both to maintaining a harmonious existence and to understanding how to redress the instabilities that can afflict us. Every substance that we encounter and every action that we perform or that is performed on us influences our inner balance for good or ill. When we adapt ourselves effectively to changing circumstances, we remain healthy; exceed our limits in any direction, and we are likely to swerve off course into the uncharted waters of illness. A full, rich, satisfying life of moderation and poise is likely to be a life that is fundamentally healthy.

What is Good Health?

The word Ayurveda can be translated in at least three different ways: "knowledge of life," "science of longevity" or "art of living." This implies that Ayurveda concentrates its activity on that difficult-to-quantify thing called "health." Ayurveda aims to train individuals to evade disease, rather than insisting that they wait for illnesses to develop before they can be treated. The Ayurvedic paradigm shows us how body, mind, and spirit interactions can be predicted, balanced, and also improved, to enable us to live gracefully, harmoniously, and vigorously. Although Ayurveda possesses many proven therapeutic techniques, its greatest treasures are these theories of health and disease.

Health is a simple concept that resists simple definition. You have probably felt it, and you know it when you see it: a woman whose step and smile and countenance radiate that certain something that feels wholesome and well nourished. To detect ill health is easy: medical textbooks are filled with its symptoms and signs. True health is a state of persistent well-being, not a condition of temporary tranquillity or a respite from affliction. Well-being is that situation in which one feels "well in one's being," a state that resists our becoming agitated or unbalanced even when circumstances may trouble or torment us. Well-being is a blend of a present-time consciousness of inner peace, calm, and stillness with an awareness of one's personal power in the context of submission to the realities of life and death—and it is also more than that.

The literal meaning of *svastha*, the Sanskrit word for "healthy," says it all: to be svastha is to be "established in yourself." Only a woman who is well established in herself will be able to radiate that joy and enthusiasm and "juiciness" of life that we recognize when we see health. In all its prescriptions and proscriptions, preventatives and remedies, Ayurveda's eye stays firmly fixed on establishing living beings within themselves.

Self-establishment requires good balance: not the dead stasis of taxidermy, but rather that dynamic equipoise in which each of an individual's constituents participates. Ayurveda seeks to generate equilibrium at all levels of a person's being—body with mind, physique with environment, personality with society—as it pursues its goal of progressively more profound states of self-integration and self-establishment.

Flow

Of all the many establishable constituents of our complex beings, what we most need to establish within ourselves is our sense of flow. Embodied life is, fundamentally, a matter of flow, for life is possible only when substances and energies continually and adroitly find their ways into and out of living organisms. Interrupt or disturb that flow sufficiently, and the being in question meets its quietus. All organisms, even those that are multi-bodied such as families, societies, and cultures, depend on healthy flow for their vitality. And, whether in a newborn child or on a circuit board, flow is healthy only when it is well channeled.

Ayurveda focuses its attention on flow, and on the canal systems that Nature has created to route our intakes and outputs on every level of existence. Some of these channels, like the digestive tract, look like tubes even to the naked eye, while others are not confined by obvious physical walls. Although the body's channels are innumerable, Ayurveda singles out the most prominent for description. Fourteen channels, which deal with the intake of nutrients, the nutrition of the tissues, the expulsion of wastes, and the mind, appear in both sexes. Two, however, appear only in female bodies: the Milk Channel, which includes all the structures and functions involved in the production of milk, and the Menstrual Channel, which encompasses everything that plays a part in the expelling of menstrual blood.

A Woman's Creativity

Although it is no easy task to define the totality of what it means to be a woman, milk and menses represent what is, from the Ayurvedic perspective, the key difference between the male and the female of our species: that of a woman's intrinsic creativity. This is neither to deny men their own creative abilities nor to suggest that women ought to do nothing but procreate quietly behind the scenes. It is a simple expression of the obvious fact that woman alone can "create" new life, that women are innately motherly. Although men can learn to "mother," it does not come naturally to them, as it does to women.

Women perpetuate the human race by creating and mothering children, they perpetuate society by creating a home that is a safe haven for those children, and they perpetuate culture by passing it on to those they mother. The health of the family, society, and culture that revolves around a woman depends to a large degree on her health, and her health rests in turn on her ability to keep her creative energies flowing. Our concern in Ayurveda is to help women find those channels, both inside and outside themselves, within which they can flow comfortably, freely, and fearlessly, so that they may best display their own innate creativity to themselves, their loved ones, and the world.

Body-Mind-Spirit

It is very easy to look for health outside ourselves, in the form of some miracle supplement or exercise routine or life partner who can provide us with what we are sure we need. What we really need to do, however, is to begin our search for good health by looking within ourselves, into the spaces we so often take for granted because they always reside within us. In the beginning of your inward quest you may see no more than you could if you were to walk from bright sunlight into a darkened room. But if you persist, your internal "eye" of perception will accommodate to your internal light, and you will then begin to "see." Each of us possesses powers for health maintenance and self-healing that we can activate if we will but learn how to let them flow.

A good way to embark on your internal search is to sit quietly in a comfortable position, your back contentedly straight and your eyes closed. Try to minimize your awareness of the external world, "look" inside instead, and try to "see" some of the principles on which the seers founded Ayurveda.

Life's Five Foundation Principles

To describe a system accurately, we need to begin by examining the principles that underlie it. Modern medical science, which has received theoretical contributions from physics, chemistry, psychology, sociology, and anthropology, among many other disciplines, has found it hard to connect these varied axioms into one unified theory of life and health. Ayurveda approaches the question from the opposite direction—from the unified to the particular. It seeks a paradigm, a systematizing model of reality that organizes life's fundamentals into a framework that the many disciplines of science and art can share.

The most central of all these fundamentals is our first axiom:

1. **Life is relationship.** No one is an island entire unto herself; every woman interacts with the world around her. All humans are dependent on food, water, light, sound, love, and other "nutrients" that flow into them from sources outside their own bodies. Each woman likewise influences that world out there, through her communications, fabrications, movements, excretions, creations, and other actions. True health requires that these many and varied flows develop a dynamic balance, an ever-changing equilibrium that propagates itself. On the physical level a woman relates to her environment, on the mental and emotional level to her society, and on the spiritual level her soul relates to Nature and Reality. Each of these relationships can be as gratifying or as tempestuous as any interpersonal relationship.

2. **The most important of all relationships is the one a woman has with herself.** Many of us look outside ourselves for our whole lives, trying to find that man (or woman), that job, that food, activity, or other object that will magically supplement our inadequacies, perfect our imperfections, and make us feel that sense of wholeness that deep down each of us craves. But nothing external to you can ever truly fill the bill, for everything that is outside you is something that can be lost. Thus the only things that you can rely on are, in the words of an ancient saying, "the things you would be able to save in a shipwreck: your body, your

mind and emotions, and your spirit." The road to health is basically a road to self-knowledge, a path of awakening to your personal realities, a melding of all your different awarenesses into one well-integrated awareness, connected at her roots to the water of life that gushes from Mother Nature's spring.

3. **A living human being is a body-mind-spirit complex.** Each part of you—organs, tissues, skeleton, nervous system, emotions, mind, and others—possesses its own form of awareness, and each of these awarenesses relates to the others. The more closely they are integrated, and the more subtle your intuitive "feel" for this integration, the better your health will be. "Mind-body" medicine is becoming popular today, driven by scientific discoveries that the endocrine, nervous, and immune systems are all closely interconnected. Every thought we have influences the body's well-being, and every chemical that enters or is created within the body affects the mind. Although mind-body medicine is a tremendous advance over the simplistic sort of mechanistic medicine that until recently has dominated the healing arts, it does not go far enough. It fails to transcend its own materialistic limits; tied down as it is to the material world, it remains ignorant of the world of spirit, of the consciousness that lies beyond matter. When we limit ourselves to the mind and body, we neglect the care of the soul. Ayurveda is the prototype of the type of healing system that the world is now slowly groping toward: body-mind-spirit medicine.

4. **Matter develops from consciousness, and an organism's consciousness continually seeks to express itself through the matter that makes up its body-mind.** Concern for soul and spirit is central to Ayurveda. India's seers discovered that consciousness is omnipresent in the universe, and that everything in the universe that is not pure, unconditional consciousness is a form of matter. The material universe and all that is within it evolved from and continues to evolve through the action of that consciousness. Consciousness expresses itself in and

through everything that exists, the variety of its expression depending on the density of the matter that contains it.

From the viewpoint of consciousness, there is nothing in the cosmos that is not consciousness. From the human point of view, however, consciousness is limited and fragmented. For one thing, it is always being interrupted. All of us must regularly exchange wakefulness for periods of dreaming and of stupor, during which our subconscious and unconscious minds will rule the mental roost. Our waking minds see one reality, our subconscious minds see another, and our unconscious minds see yet another. Even the individual cells of our bodies possess their own individual awarenesses, which combine into tissue- and organ-perceptions that, when taken together, represent a "whole-body" comprehension. But the sum of all these comprehensions still remains a mosaic, a patchwork of discrete awarenesses that are all individually reflecting that One Reality of seamless, attribute-free consciousness.

This concept of consciousness is, of course, diametrically opposed to that of modern materialist science, which teaches that consciousness evolved from matter. And although the Ayurvedic position cannot yet be conclusively "proved," scientific evidence of consciousness's ability to influence matter, at least in the form of observers affecting their observations, continues to accumulate. In his book *Healing Words*, Larry Dossey, M.D., comments on one recent advance: "It appears that double-blind studies can sometimes be steered in directions that correspond to the thoughts and attitudes of the experimenters. This might shed light on why skeptical experimenters appear unable to replicate the findings of believers, and why 'true believers' seem more able to produce positive results. The validity of decades of experimental findings in medical research would need to be reevaluated if it is proved that the mind can 'shove the data around.'"

Ayurveda's seers long pondered the ways in which humans shove their data around. They studied how a living being's physical body, *prana* (life force), thinking mind, emotional mind, and consciousness interplay within the functional relationships that exist between that being and its environment. One group of such observations centers around prana. This life force, which the Chinese call *chi* and the Japanese *ki*, can be described as the energy that inspires life to persist within a particular body-mind-spirit complex. Prana is therefore the *shakti* (energy) of the body-mind-spirit complex; it invigorates and inspires the body, transports the mind wherever it needs to go, and aligns the soul's awareness with that of the Absolute Spirit. Those students of yoga, tai chi, and the martial arts who learn to identify and circulate this force within themselves discover that prana is easily measured with internal instruments.

5. **All flows in all parts of an organism interact with and influence one another.** People who learn to locate and gauge prana soon realize that wherever the mind flows there will flow the prana, and she who can direct her prana to one of her limbs or organs will find her mind directed there as well. Her experiments will soon convince her, however, that all flows are not equal. In fact, the flow of influence is predominantly from subtler to denser. Prana is subtler than the body, hence changes in the flow of prana will ordinarily affect the body more than changes in the body will affect prana. Mind being subtler than prana, its influence on prana is usually more significant than in the reverse direction; and when we bare our souls to ourselves we will find them instigating the mind far more efficiently than the mind, or prana, or body can motivate the soul.

   Soul and *spirit* are concepts that have been out of fashion for so long in the West that they are unfamiliar to many of us. We can use the word *soul* to represent that portion of spirit which is our personal parcel of consciousness, that sentience which supplies our awareness. We can call unqualified, unlimited consciousness *spirit,* which makes spirituality the progressive awakening of our limited souls to the infinity of possibilities present in the theater of the Absolute.

Two

HEALTH, DISEASE, AND THE THREE DOSHAS

The *Charaka Samhita* states boldly that no doctor has ever been or will ever be able to create and maintain health. Nature alone can heal and provide health. All that a human can do is to create conditions in herself or her patients that will facilitate Nature's work.

Health and Consciousness

The ultimate in healing is to attune a body-mind-spirit complex so finely to the universal consciousness that that consciousness begins to direct the organism's functions. The individual can then grow into a state of harmony with each and every flow in the universe. Ayurveda's seers did just this: they developed unprecedented states of balance in themselves through their profoundly intuitive ability to align themselves with the Absolute. Although few will ever attain such subtlety of awareness, each of us can strive to maximize the manifestation of consciousness within ourselves, in all its various forms. Consciousness is everywhere—it is just a matter of awakening it and allowing it to transform you. Each level of experience possesses its own intelligence, and you will know you have embarked on the journey toward true health when you have introduced yourself to the varied intelligences of your mind, body, prana, emotions, and soul. You will have to leave your rational mind behind when you commune with the parts of your organism that are not "rational," however: "consciousnessness" and "rationality" are two very different things.

Consciousness, properly applied, is without doubt the best of all medicines, provided that it is available to you. Unfortunately, conditions are such in our world (and in ourselves, since we live in relationship with our world) that imbalances may develop which resist all but the most vigorous of physical treatments, such as surgery, radiation, or chemotherapy. "The medicine is that which cures the disease," says Ayurveda, whose philosophy proposes both that we use the simplest therapy in order to treat an illness and that we never hesitate to attack disease aggressively when nothing but aggression will suffice to preserve life. The more boundaries that exist within you, the less freely your consciousness—and your mind, your prana, and the substances within your body—will be able to flow. These are the constraints that will limit your health. The better you can awaken your awareness, the better you will flow through life, and the more health will accrue to you.

We humans live in an imperfect world because we are by nature imperfect. Those of us who seek to work our way into states of enhanced health will do well to begin with our most limited state of consciousness, which happens to be the physical body. A strong, healthy body provides a stable foundation upon which sound structures of consciousness can be erected. In Ayurveda we study the physical body both directly, by examining and seeking to learn how to manipulate its tissues and wastes, and indirectly, by investigating the forces which control it.

The Three Doshas

Ayurveda's seers isolated three forces which are particularly important, because they permit us to understand associations that exist between seemingly unconnected causal pathways and manifested symptoms within an organism. These forces are called the three doshas. The word *dosha* means "fault," "mistake," "imperfection," although the doshas are paradoxically forces that both preserve an organism's balance and rhythm when they are themselves balanced, yet will disturb its harmony when they are disturbed. Like prana, these three doshas are invisible forces which cannot be directly perceived. Only their actions can be demonstrated, through the bodily substances which are their vehicles. These include (but are not limited to) nervous impulses for vata, bile for pitta, and mucus for kapha.

These three doshas are condensations of the five *mahabhutas*—the five "great elements"—more properly known as the five "great states of material existence." They are:

1. **Earth.** The solid state of matter, the characteristic attribute of which is stability.

2. **Water.** The liquid state of matter, whose characteristic attribute is flux.

3. **Fire.** The power that can convert a substance from solid to liquid to gas, or vice versa.

4. **Air.** The gaseous state of matter, whose characteristic attribute is mobility.

5. **Space.** The field from which everything is manifested and into which everything returns; the space in which events occur. Space (which can also be translated as "ether") has no perceptible physical existence. It appears in our world as the distances that separate matter.

In the context of a living organism's physiology, the force that shows the greatest influence of the air is vata. Pitta shows the greatest influence of fire, and kapha of water.

    Vata, the body's principle of kinetic energy, is in charge of all motion in the body and mind.

    Kapha, the principle of potential energy, is the stabilizing influence in the living being; it also lubricates and maintains.

- Pitta, which is in charge of all transformation in the organism, controls the balance of its kinetic and potential energies.

The three doshas pervade the body, working in every cell at every instant, but they concentrate themselves in those tissues in which they are particularly required:

- Vata is particularly active in the brain and nervous system, the heart, colon, bones, lungs, bladder, pelvis, thighs, ears, and skin.

- Pitta concentrates in the brain, liver, spleen, small intestine, endocrine glands, skin, eyes, blood, and sweat.

- Kapha is most prevalent in the brain, joints, mouth, head and neck, stomach, lymph, thorax (especially lungs, heart, and esophagus) and fat.

Each of the doshas has five varieties, or subdoshas. Although these subdoshas tend to act as if they were distinct entities, they are merely specializations of the three doshas, created by Nature to perform specific tasks.

- The five kaphas are manifest in body lubricants, including stomach mucus, pleural and pericardial fluid, saliva, synovial fluid, and cerebrospinal fluid.

- The five pittas appear in transformative substances, including the digestive juices, hemoglobin, melanin, rhodopsin, and various neurotransmitters.

- The five vatas divide the body into spheres of influence according to the direction of their motion: forward and back in the chest, upward in the head, circular in the digestive tract, outward and inward in the periphery, and downward in the pelvis.

Even though they are imperceptible to our senses, the three doshas are still forms of matter. They are more conscious matter than is the matter that makes up the body, which allows them to influence the body efficiently, and they are less conscious than prana, the thinking mind, and the emotions. These higher structures can therefore efficiently control the doshas—but only in those people who have carefully aligned their prana, thinking mind, and emotions with the higher consciousness of the soul and the spirit. Others tend to align their awarenesses with what is going on in their bodies—which allows them to fall prey to imbalance of the dosha forces.

Vata, pitta, and kapha are "waste products" created during the subtle metabolism of the higher forces that are prana and its associates, *tejas* (the universal fire that discriminates and digests, also called *agni*) and *ojas* (the subtle glue that integrates body, mind, and spirit together into a functioning individual). Like urine, feces, and sweat, the three doshas support the body only as long as they flow out of it continuously. In fact, proper elimination of these physical wastes helps to maintain healthy levels of the doshas within the body: urine is a vehicle for removing the kapha force, sweat carries away excess pitta force, and defecation expels excess vata force. When

QUALITIES		
Vata	Pitta	Kapha
dry	oily	oily
cold	hot	cold
light	light	heavy
irregular	intense	stable
mobile	fluid	viscous
rarefied	malodorous	dense
rough	liquid	smooth

an organism is healthy, little waste is produced; when it is in poor health, waste will accumulate. This is one of the main reasons why those who possess good health tend to amass more of it, and those who are sick will usually get sicker until they change their ways.

Like all other substances, the three doshas also possess qualities, and their increase or decrease in your system depends upon the similar or antagonistic qualities of everything you ingest—physically, energetically, mentally, emotionally, and spiritually.

All substances and all activities increase and decrease the three doshas according to their qualities. In particular, it is almost always the case that anything dry increases vata, anything hot increases pitta, and anything heavy increases kapha, for vata is the only dry dosha, pitta the only hot dosha, and kapha the only heavy dosha. If we wished to express this reality in awareness terms, we might say that vata communicates dryness to the organism, that pitta's message to a person is heat, and finally, that kapha proclaims heaviness throughout the being.

Constitution

One of the truly amazing things about life is how easy it is for an impermanent organism to project an illusion of permanence by maintaining a stable form. Molecules and atoms may come and go, but the body goes on and on. Who you are today depends on who you were yesterday, and who you will become tomorrow depends on what you make of yourself today. The disadvantage to this stability of person and personality, however, is the resistance that it produces in us to changing our ways. Our physical and mental habits benefit us to the extent that they promote good health; to the extent that they promote imbalance, they are our bane.

Personal Constitution

Ayurveda teaches that each individual possesses certain characteristic physical and mental traits that are fixed at the moment of conception and persist throughout that individual's existence. We call this pattern the personal constitution (in Sanskrit, *prakriti*), which we distinguish from *vikriti*, the changeable current state of a person's health which is her temporary condition. Your constitution is your personal metabolic make-up, your set of metabolic tendencies that determine how your body and mind will instinctively react when confronted by a stimulus. Many of the traits you prize in your personality, and many of those you dislike in yourself, develop from these tendencies. To know the inherent strengths and weaknesses of your constitution allows you to understand better how your body-mind-spirit complex functions, and how you can use diet and lifestyle changes to influence your health.

Your constitution is expressed in terms of the three doshas, because it is through the medium of the doshas that these patterns and tendencies display themselves. Some people are "uni-doshic": they naturally display the characteristics of one of the doshas so strongly that we can say that dosha rules them constitutionally. Other people are "bi-doshic": that is, one dosha predominates in them, but a second dosha is strong enough to be significantly influential in their lives on a regular basis. A few people are "tri-doshic" in a negative way: all three of their doshas are equally likely to go out of balance. A selected few are "tri-doshic" in a positive way: they are constitutionally so well balanced that no one dosha can show any particular predominance. Most of us, however, are "bi-doshic": the one dosha that influences us most strongly is followed closely by a second dosha whose effect is almost as pronounced.

If, for example, your constitution is vata-pitta, throughout your life you will be prone to over-activity of both vata and pitta. Imbalances may come and go, but when your system is stressed it will always be more likely that either vata or pitta, or both, will initially go out of balance. Your constitution is your first reaction to stress, and from the point of view of your body-mind-spirit, any need to adapt acts as a stress. The need to adapt is universal, but the ways in which people adapt differ from person to person. Many of these adaptation patterns are learned behavior, but others are innate properties of the organism itself. Everyone has physical, psychological, pranic, and emotional strengths and weaknesses which, taken together, form a set of "reaction prints" that are as characteristic of their owners as are fingerprints or footprints. The aggregate of these innate properties forms your personal constitution—the temperament which profoundly influences predisposition to health, general and specific sensitivity to illness, and responsiveness to various forms of therapy.

Energy Flow

Your constitutional type is an expression of your organism's energy-flow strategy, in all realms of existence.

⁂ Vata people make active use of their energy, spending it freely and frequently wasting it, because vata is governed by kinetic energy, the energy of action. Vata exerts a cold, dry, irregular influence on a system, because this dosha encourages energy to be expended as soon as it enters the organism.

⁂ Kapha types are governed by potential energy, which gives them a genetic predisposition to save and steward energy well.

⁂ Pitta manages energies of all sorts, and produces a hot, oily, and irritable effect because this dosha must maintain a high level of reactivity in order to manipulate energy effectively.

⁂ Pitta pushes your channels in the direction of dilation, kapha promotes channel congestion, and vata encourages them to constrict (while channels affected by vata usually fluctuate readily and rapidly between dilation and constriction, they tend to end up in the constricted mode).

Constitutional Strategy

Your organism will tend to favor your constitutional strategy whenever it is exposed to a stimulus to which it must respond. For example, everyone will feel cold during the winter, but vata people usually feel colder sooner than do pitta people, and their hands and feet feel colder longer. Pitta's dilating power encourages blood to flow through the channels that are the arteries, thereby warming the chilled limbs. Vata thus communicates "coolness" and pitta "heat" to the body-mind-spirit. Pitta people commonly feel more hunger sooner than do kapha types, because the pitta digestive fire is always being stimulated by the movement of digestive juices in the dilated digestive channel. This is one of the ways in which pitta produces "heat" within an organism. Pitta hunger may announce itself as hunger for food, for some other sort of physical gratification, for achievement, or as some other sort of appetite. In every context in life pitta notifies us of heat, which makes for hunger. Kapha speaks to us of slowness, solidity, and relaxation, and one of the media through which it expresses itself is body weight. Accordingly, kapha people tend to gain weight more easily and lose it with more difficulty than do other types; their systems are engineered to store matter and energy, and will automatically do so when the opportunity arises unless some corrective is applied. Many vata people, who often find it difficult to retain either matter or energy, envy kapha people because of their pronounced tendency to retain both. Pitta people have a knack for managing both well and they usually get into trouble by over-managing themselves.

Assessing Your Constitution

Given the various possible combinations of the three doshas, the number of constitutional types is truly as infinite as the number of possible individuals. There are, however, eight main groups of constitutional types. Of these, six are most common: vata, pitta, and kapha each predominating alone; and vata-pitta or pitta-vata, pitta-kapha or kapha-pitta, and vata-kapha or kapha-vata predominating together. Those individuals in whom all three doshas tend toward imbalance are rarely able to be truly healthy, while those rare individuals in whom the three doshas tend always to remain in balance usually remain healthy so effortlessly that they have to be severely stressed before any sort of imbalance develops.

Your personal constitution was determined by the state of the bodies of your mother and father at the time of your conception, modified by your parents' genetics, your mother's diet and habits during her pregnancy, and any abnormal events at the time of your birth. Once your personal constitution and its accompanying tendencies have been set, however, they cannot be permanently altered. Like it or not, you have your constitution for the rest of your life. Until then, you will have to rely on knowing your own personal constitution in order to develop effective strategies for creating and maintaining the balance that is good health. Understanding your constitution helps you to understand why you do the things you do, and what you can do to improve yourself.

Determining your constitution is not difficult, unless you happen to be so strongly swayed by it that you have developed a distorted perspective. This is not uncommon: vata people often believe it is normal to have lots of nervous energy, pitta people tend to believe that it is normal to be driven, and many kapha people prefer to believe that inertia is normal. That the doshas can make us believe that abnormality is normal is yet more evidence of the pervasive bias they devise in our lives.

When you try to determine your own constitution, you should evaluate yourself as accurately and honestly as you can, without being tempted to see yourself as you would like to be. It may be educational to have a friend evaluate you as well, and then compare the two.

You should respond to the questionnaire below according to how you have reacted in general throughout your entire lifetime. Select the description that fits you most accurately overall. Whenever things have changed greatly during your life, vata is the appropriate answer, even if the vata description in that category does not accurately describe you as you are today. Also select vata whenever you are confused about your answer. Select all responses that apply to you; you will find that you have some amount of each dosha in your constitution.

As you are evaluating yourself, keep in mind that:

- Vata is cold, dry, and irregular.

- Pitta is hot, oily, and irritable.

- Kapha is cold, wet, and stable.

CONSTITUTION QUESTIONNAIRE

ॐ VATA

Physical Assessment

☐ I am slim and lanky without much muscular definition.

☐ It is difficult for me to gain weight.

☐ My skin is cool, rough, and dry.

☐ My hair is dark, curly, and dry.

☐ My eyes are small and dark brown, gray, or slate blue.

Physical Tendencies

☐ I prefer warm weather.

☐ My energy is inconsistent and usually comes in bursts.

☐ I am active but I lose stamina quickly.

☐ My physical stamina is often poor.

☐ I do not usually require much sleep, and I sleep lightly.

☐ I am talkative.

☐ My appetite is irregular.

☐ My elimination is irregular, alternating between dry and loose stools, and I am prone to constipation.

Temperament Assessment

☐ I learn new things easily, but I tend to forget easily, as well.

☐ I tend be nervous or anxious.

☐ My moods fluctuate, often unpredictably.

☐ I am creative and imaginative. I like to express myself creatively.

☐ My thoughts are often dreams which I do not see through to their fruition.

☐ I lead an erratic lifestyle.

✤ PITTA

Physical Assessment

☐ I am of medium physique with good muscular development.

☐ I gain and lose weight fairly easily.

☐ My skin is warm and may be oily.

☐ My hair is light, straight, and fine.

☐ My eyes are sharp, lustrous, and bright blue or light brown.

Physical Tendencies

☐ I prefer cool weather.

☐ My energy level is moderate.

☐ I enjoy physical activity and sweat easily.

☐ I enjoy average stamina.

☐ I require a moderate amount of sleep, and I sleep soundly.

☐ I am assertive when talking, and I have a strong voice.

☐ My appetite is good, and I need to eat regularly.

☐ My elimination is regular, with soft stools that tend to be loose.

☐ My food moves through me quickly.

Temperament Assessment

☐ My memory is good and quick.

☐ I tend to anger easily, and to become impatient and irritated.

☐ My moods take a back seat to my goals and tasks.

☐ I am efficient, organized, and I am a perfectionist.

☐ My thoughts and ideas are logical and well planned.

☐ I lead a busy lifestyle.

☀ KAPHA

Physical Assessment
- ☐ I am of large, rounded, build with good muscular development.
- ☐ It is difficult for me to lose weight.
- ☐ My skin is cool, smooth, and moist.
- ☐ My hair is thick, wavy, and may be light or dark.
- ☐ My eyes are large, attractive, and brown.

Physical Tendencies
- ☐ I enjoy all climates, but I prefer warm weather.
- ☐ My energy level is steady.
- ☐ Although I tend to be lethargic, I have good endurance.
- ☐ My physical strength is good.
- ☐ I like to sleep, and I sleep deeply.
- ☐ I talk slowly, with a pleasant, resonant voice.
- ☐ My appetite is steady, I eat slowly, and I enjoy food.
- ☐ My elimination is regular, and my food moves through me slowly.

Temperament Assessment
- ☐ I learn new things slowly, but once learned they are rarely forgotten.
- ☐ I tend to be calm, steady, and possessive.
- ☐ I am caring and compassionate.
- ☐ My thoughts and ideas are tranquil and well organized.
- ☐ I am thorough and good at following through on tasks.
- ☐ I have a relaxed and slow-paced lifestyle.

The summaries below may help you confirm your evaluation of your own constitution:

Vata predominant

Vata people do things quickly, and change quickly. Some days they are full of energy, their digestion is good, and they sleep well, while on others they drag themselves through the day, can't figure out what to eat, and sleep like colicky babies. Their bodies and minds tend toward restlessness, and their energy comes in spurts. They tend to use up their energy on the things to which they are addicted, then have to wait impatiently for more energy to accumulate once that store is spent. The vata body tends to be dry, rough, and cold, and the vata mind imaginative; fear or anxiety is vata's predominant negative emotion. If changeability characterizes most of what you do, then you are vata predominant. Because of its spendthrift ways with matter and energy, the vata constitution is the most difficult to keep in good health.

Pitta predominant

Pitta people are mentally and physically efficient, precise and orderly, which can make them feel obligated to offer pointed criticisms of themselves and others. They tend to hate heat unless they have become addicted to its stimulation, and their warm, soft, freckled or pimpled skin tends to react poorly to heat and to the sun. Strong-mindedly forceful, they often try to impose their will on others, whether consciously or unconsciously. They love to eat and to compete, and usually become irritated by disagreement and hunger, and impatient with those who are slower on the uptake than they. They can become so focused on whatever it is they do well that they may sacrifice everything else in order to be successful at it. Their natural heat creates courage when it is well disciplined, and anger otherwise. Heat, physical and mental, creates most of their diseases. If you apply intensity and competitiveness to almost everything you do, you are pitta predominant.

Kapha predominant

Kapha people, who like the slow, relaxed life, are solidly built individuals who gain weight easily and lose it with difficulty unless they exercise regularly. Their bodies are usually well nourished, they normally sleep deeply, and they commonly prefer to eat, walk, and talk slowly. They may also learn slowly, but they rarely forget. They are prone to congestion, but possess superior stamina and can skip meals without physical discomfort. Underneath their calm exteriors they are often strongly emotional beings. They tend to be complacent, and may be averse even to needed change. Kapha is the constitutional type that, properly maintained, remains healthy with the least effort. If slow but steady is your watchword, both physically and mentally, then you are likely to be kapha predominant.

Reacting to Stimuli

Pitta promotes warmth, appetite, and desire by dilating an organism's channels. Vata and kapha consume warmth, vata by radiating it away with activity and kapha by mopping it up with matter. When vata dries up a being's juices, pitta and kapha replenish them, and when kapha weighs a body down, pitta or vata is ready to lighten and reactivate it. The three doshas work by mutual suppression, each trying its best to outshine the others. In the healthy body-mind-spirit, the three are so well balanced that none becomes paramount; in imbalance one begins to dictate terms to the others. Sometimes imbalances are created by acts of commission: by eating too many of the foods, or by doing too many of the things, and thinking too many of the thoughts that empower one or other of the doshas. Other imbalances, however, arise from omission, that is, from failing to compensate for the influence of one of the natural cyclic changes that form Nature's constitution.

Your constitution is a measurement of your body-mind-spirit's potential to react to stimuli. How much of that potential will be activated depends on the nature of the trigger. Every quality of every substance with which you come in contact, and every action that you perform or that is performed on you, will empower or inhibit one or more of your doshas. In order to try to predict just how substances and actions might influence you and your organism, we need to know both the nature and intensity of the quality that influences you, and the nature and intensity of your response.

Seasons

One of the strongest determinants of intensity, both in the thing that affects you and the degree to which you are affected by it, will be the season in which it occurs.

The rhythm of waxing and waning, of dilation and contraction, is central to embodied life. Our internal peristaltic waves, brain waves and thought waves are all intricately interrelated with one another and with our external environments. Plants and animals, which have no conscious time sense, have Nature to keep them "in sync" with the seasons. We humans, though, are on our own, to the extent that we have traded away our instincts for the conscious use of our senses. This forces those of us who wish to live healthily to synchronize ourselves actively with Nature's rhythms.

Ayurveda recognizes four main "seasonal" cycles that apply to men and women alike. Establishing a rhythm in each of these cycles is essential to continued physical health, for it helps you to flow in the direction that is most appropriate for you.

I. Day and Night

From dawn to mid-morning kapha predominates, as the system is stimulated into activity by wakefulness and sunlight. Mid-morning to mid-afternoon is pitta time, when heat and concentrated action predominate both in the environment and in the organisms that inhabit it. After this crest comes the out-of-focus period from mid-afternoon to dusk, during which the vata force progressively increases. Vata's power maximizes at dusk, after which kapha predominates from dusk through slightly more than the first one-third of the night. Pitta rules the midnight hours, and vata accumulates through the pre-dawn hours until it reaches its other daily culmination at dawn.

When we look at the twenty-four hours as a whole, we find that pitta predominates during the day, which is warmer than the night, when kapha predominates. Vata again owns dawn and dusk, the junctions of day and night. Layered on top of these cycles is yet another: the cycle of breathing. We breathe through only one nostril at a time, our nostrils switching on and off roughly every ninety minutes. The action of the left nostril is to cool and calm the body-mind-spirit, which may enhance kapha's force; the right nostril heats and agitates the system, which can magnify pitta. When both nostrils work together it is possible for vata to increase, and this happens naturally only around the times of sunrise and sunset—vata's natural times of day.

2. Seasons of the Year

The year's seasons differ from climate to climate, but in most of the temperate countries kapha accumulates during the winter and can become obstructive in spring; pitta accumulates during spring to become dictatorial in summer, when kapha wanes; and vata, which waxes during the summer, climaxes in autumn, when pitta calms itself. Vata then gradually calms itself during winter as kapha begins to collect itself again.

3. Digestion

Immediately after you eat, the mass of food you have ingested causes kapha to predominate and pitta to increase. During digestion pitta predominates, kapha calms down, and vata accumulates. Pitta cools off and vata works hardest after digestion, when nutrients are assimilated and wastes excreted.

4. Lifespan

Kapha rules a girl from birth until the time she reaches full development. Thereafter it takes a back seat to pitta until age thirty-five or so, while integration of body and mind progresses. Pitta's sway is unchallenged from then until menopause, after which vata's strength increases. Vata accelerates after age sixty, as the body-mind-spirit complex gradually disintegrates.

The Menstrual Cycle

Women enjoy an extra season, the menstrual cycle. Actually both sexes have an "endocrine" season, but a man's, which is still poorly understood, appears to be based on the sun instead of the moon (a man's testosterone, for example, reaches a peak in spring and bottoms out in autumn). Most women who are in touch with their emotions seem to find greater interest in sexual activity during the period surrounding the full moon. Although there are scientists who strenuously maintain that it is only coincidence that the menstrual cycle lasts precisely as long as the lunar cycle, Indian tradition holds that women enjoy a special relationship with the moon. In fact, it is generally agreed that ideally a woman ovulates with the full moon, when the heavens encourage her body and mind to be plump and juicy. She optimally menstruates with the new moon, which is encouraging her body to expel unused fertility juices.

The menstrual cycle is itself strongly influenced by the three doshas. Thus in a healthy woman, kapha will increase during her proliferative phase, which lasts from the end of her flow until ovulation. Estrogen, in many ways a kapha-like hormone, should peak during this stage. Progesterone, a more pitta-type hormone, takes over predominance from estrogen during the secretory phase, which lasts from ovulation until the flow begins. Pitta then predominates in the woman's body during this second half of the month. Vata, whose task in the organism is transport, dominates during the days of flow, as it transports the menstrual blood out of the body.

Preventing Disease

Ayurveda tells us that diseases are generated at the junctions of the seasons, the moments when one season changes into another. Whenever our environment (internal or external) changes, our systems must change with it, and every time we adapt poorly we expose ourselves to the possibility of disease. Dawn and dusk are the "joints" of day and night, ovulation and menstruation are the joints of the menstrual cycle, and menarche and menopause are the junctions of a woman's life. A general Sanskrit term for the menstrual cycle and the substances associated with it is *artava*, a word which is derived from *rtu*, meaning season.

The quest for good health requires daily and seasonal routine activities to prevent illness, purificatory and palliative therapies to relieve it, and rejuvenation to enhance health and quality of life. Even serious imbalances such as autoimmune disease, cancer, and heart disease can undoubtedly benefit from the integrated approach to health that is Ayurveda—although it is much better to prevent illness before it occurs, and to avert miseries that have not yet arrived.

Preventive medicine, which is based on individual constitution, is called in Ayurveda *svastha vritta*, "establishing oneself in good habits." It teaches the rejection of excess in everything, for harmony and health can develop only when we enjoy the things in our lives in the proper amount and at the proper moment.

Regular seasonal purifications, which form one segment of preventive medicine, are prescribed to everyone in Ayurveda to help protect against potential ailments at the seasonal joints. For example, to protect against imbalances that might arise from inattention to the ceaseless turning of the day's seasons, Ayurveda prescribes a daily routine. While each routine is tailored to the individual who will be performing it, the average routine begins at or before dawn, when one rises to eliminate urine and feces. Metabolic wastes are then mobilized and expelled through massage and exercise, external wastes of all kinds are dislodged by bathing, and mental wastes are purged by meditation.

Each season of the year has a purification regimen appropriate to the doshas which it threatens to engender within us. Generally speaking, excess kapha should be expelled in spring—for instance, by fasting for one or several days (depending on your constitution, condition, and strength) and drinking weak ginger tea or some similar substance. Summer is the pitta-ejecting time, for which aloe vera (up to two ounces twice a day) can be beneficial. When autumn comes around vata should be reduced by consuming roots (as vegetables, decoctions, or herbal supplements), oil massage, and sometimes oil enema. A competent Ayurvedic physician can design a regimen of seasonal purification to fit your personal requirements.

Your Creative Potential

Menstruation is itself a seasonal purification—a way women's bodies and minds have of purifying themselves each month. Nature provides women with this service for her own purposes, of course. She wants healthy children, to which end there is no substitute for healthy mothers. A wise woman will work with Nature to take advantage of this natural monthly cleansing, so that both she and Nature can achieve their goals. Nature does not want you to become pregnant each month; she does not even insist that you become pregnant at all. She does request, though, that your body and mind remain in regular contact with their roots, in that creativity which females alone possess. Nature is happy for you to use your formative ability in any way you feel fit—for yourself or for others, to generate or to repair, to create or procreate. She becomes so pleased when you use that power to assist others, whether those others belong to you or not, that she will contribute her own power to you to add to your own creativity. When you cut yourself off from your wellspring, you block Nature's efforts to help and heal you—and this blockage will often display itself most vividly as some impediment to your menstrual flow.

Because a healthy physical creative potential is so important to a woman's healthy life flow, this book is organized around the three seasons of a woman's life that fertility creates: the premenstrual moment of childhood, the menstrual years of adulthood, and the postmenstrual time of wisdom.

Three

CHILDHOOD
THE KAPHA AGE

The relationship that you evolve with the world around you has its roots in the relationship that develops between your personal constitution (prakriti), which is your innate nature, and your surroundings. From the moment of your conception, the flavor and texture of your experience of life is influenced by everything that your mother eats, drinks, does and thinks while you swim in her womb, and by how your parents relate to one another before, during, and after your genesis. The qualities of the environment into which you plunge at birth continue this already on-going process. Your nature and your nurture work together, in varying degrees, during your formative years to produce the "you" that you become.

Ideally, every experience that you have as a fetus, as an infant, and as a young girl will be of the sustaining, confidence-producing variety, for this sort will allow you to ripen into the perception that the outside world is intrinsically benevolent (or, at the least, not malicious). When a child is repeatedly confronted with situations that disturb her sense of security or self-worth, undesirable patterns arise in her metabolism and mind which may prove remarkably resistant to later resolution. Children who are misshapen early on tend, like bent saplings, to retain their bends even after they are permitted to grow straight.

Taste

Every sort of stimulus encourages or discourages its own metabolite or neurotransmitter within the body, and when one variety of stimulus is repeated frequently the organism becomes conditioned by it. When significantly strong, that conditioning can determine the organism's state. We might say, for example, that arousing aggression in a child again and again may cause it to develop an internal tendency to over-produce the substance norepinephrine and under-produce serotonin, leading to a state of near-permanent nervous alarm.

In Ayurveda, we express relations between metabolism and emotion in terms of "taste" instead of chemicals. Most of us do not rely on chemical analysis to determine whether a piece of fruit is palatable; our taste buds tell us that, instantly and reliably. Nor should we expect biochemistry to be able to "quantify" sensations like your personal "flavor," which can be effectively analyzed by quality alone. What Ayurvedic analysis sacrifices in quantitative detail it makes up for in the qualitative particularization of your life's "flavor," which is a synopsis of your experiences of the mental and physical "sap" that you create within yourself via your reactions to the stimuli that you absorb. This flavor permeates your existence and your consciousness, making your personality sour or salty, your existence bitter or sweet. This flavor is the reality in which you live your life, the factor which contributes mightily to making your life blissful, miserable, or something in between.

Everything in a landscape, be it the external environment in which we live or the internal environment of the human organism, is permeated by flavor. The most common Sanskrit word used for flavor is *rasa*, a word that encompasses everything that is "juicy" in one's existence. Lymph and blood plasma, semen, milk and other tissue juices, fruit and vegetable juices, and soups are all rasas, or "fluid realities." Rasa also indicates the sense of taste, and one's emotions. The flavors of the juices that make up our bodies and minds, derived both from what we imbibe from without and generate within, combine to create our personal emotional rasas, the subjective perceptions that are the juices that water your soul.

Diet

The sun "cooks" water and soil nutrients into plants, whose sap takes on a particular flavor which can be tasted by every organism that possesses a taste sense. The organisms that eat these plants take on their flavors, and when these organisms are eaten by a human being, that person acquires their taste qualities. The emotion you bring to your table will help to determine how well or poorly you digest and assimilate these flavors, and each of the flavors you consume will augment, alter, or diminish the quality and intensity of your various emotions.

While both your physical rasa (derived from the juices and tastes that appear in your food) and your mental rasa (derived from your emotions) contribute to the overall "flavor" of your person, the most important influence on your "juices," particularly in childhood, is your diet. A child is growing, continually laying down physical and mental structures on which she will rely for the remainder of her existence. Food is a child's construction material, her bricks and mortar. By delivering tastes along with protein, carbohydrate and fat, each morsel of food nourishes both her physique and her emotions.

Ayurveda teaches that the taste of food is itself nutritious to an organism; as you eat, so you become. When you consciously select appropriate tastes in the food, drink, medicine, activity, climate, seasons, and other "substances" that you take in, the juices that your body-mind-spirit produces after digestion will be sweet, which will make you satisfied and happy. "Sweetness" is the emotion that everyone pursues, whether she is aware of it or not. When your internal space is filled with sweet juice it attracts external sweetness to it, and life's harmony multiplies. Food is not our only source of sweetness, but it is one of the most crucial. A healthy life only develops from the sort of healthy flow that healthy food provides.

The Six Tastes

While "sweetness" the emotion is promoted by "sweet" the taste, obviously a diet of sugar alone would be unhealthy. "Sweet" is therefore valuable only in the context of the other members of the group of six tastes which interchange to create your organism's flavor. These six tastes apply to each sense organ, but they are called "tastes" because their most important influence is on the make-up of the juices of our bodies and minds.

A few exceptional people find all the bliss they need within themselves; those who cannot must extract most of the tastes they require from their environments. What tastes we take will determine which doshas we reinforce. A kapha-type individual who takes in

THE SIX TASTES	
SWEET	Cold, oily, and heavy; increases kapha and reduces vata and pitta.
SOUR	Hot, oily, and light; increases kapha and pitta, and reduces vata.
SALTY	Hot, oily, and heavy; like sour, it increases kapha and pitta, and reduces vata.
PUNGENT	The spicy taste, which is hot, dry, and light; increases vata and pitta, and reduces kapha.
BITTER	Cold, dry, and light; increases vata, and reduces pitta and kapha.
ASTRINGENT	Cold, dry, and heavy; increases vata, and reduces pitta and kapha.

tastes that promote kapha accumulation will find it much more dif-ficult to stay well than will a similar kapha individual who eats food that contains tastes which balance kapha. Pitta people do better with pitta-calming than with pitta-inflaming tastes, and a vata per-son will do well to pursue a diet high in vata-controlling rather than vata-inflating tastes.

Since sweet happens to be kapha's predominant taste, and kapha happens to dominate in children, children are naturally sweet and naturally attract sweetness to them, particularly while they live on milk alone, which is sweet. After a child begins to eat, her constitutional preferences help to determine what foods she will be attracted to. Under ordinary conditions, a healthy child will eat what her body wants to eat, because she allows her body to decide her diet for her. A child's innate food preferences can tell her parents quite a lot about her constitution, if they happen to be paying attention.

Toxins: Ama

A child who has been diverted from her natural preferences at an early age will often start to follow the promptings of her abnormal patterns instead of her body, and will seek out foods that will help perpetuate those patterns. Taste preferences and aversions acquired when you are young have a habit of persisting, and can mean the difference between a lifelong tendency to health and a persistent trend to imbalance. The dangers of becoming addicted to sweets are very well known, but how many people know of the hazards of a salt or sour or spice addiction? Or that overeating protein, which requires calcium for its metabolism, can rob the bones of some of the calcium they will need later in life to prevent osteoporosis? (There is more about osteoporosis on page 137.)

Food is of particular importance to children because the stomach is the body's seat of kapha, and many of the maladies that beset chil-dren originate there. The body uses an upset tummy to signal its indignation over a food it cannot use and so refuses to accept. Under normal circumstances, this sort of negative conditioning encourages children to move away from foods that don't agree with them.

But we are not living under normal circumstances when billions of dollars are being spent on advertising to encourage all of us to eat what is not good for us. When the U.S. government can declare ketchup a vegetable (during the Reagan administration), it is tempting to conclude that a conspiracy exists to strip our children of their nutritional rights. The occasional fast-food foray is rarely permanently detrimental, but daily consumption of pizza, burgers, and greasy chips can be. Although the body will continue to announce its ire periodically with indigestion, when under continual junk food onslaught it will begin to absorb some of the toxic material that its mouth is wolfing down. In fact, even the healthiest food can produce toxins when it is eaten, if the digestive capacity is already weakened or the mind and emotions are under significant stress. Any time your body-mind-spirit system becomes unbalanced it is possible that the food (physical, mental, emotional, energetic) you eat will be improperly digested. The toxins that result are collectively called *ama* in Ayurveda.

Ama produces a child's upset tummy, and it is also to blame for most of the disturbances that young flesh is heir to. Simple fevers are usually due to ama, as are most varieties of respiratory congestion. Even bronchial asthma is regarded in Ayurveda as being "born from the stomach." Ama and kapha are very similar in quality, which makes children particularly prone to invasion by these toxins. If a child's urine is turbid with a foul odor, or her feces sticky, full of pieces of undigested food, offensive in odor, and passed with abundant gas, ama is present. A thick and unpleasant-looking coating on her tongue also testifies to ama in her digestive tract, particularly if her breath smells rank or "unripe."

When invaded by ama, a child automatically loses her appetite and will not find it again until the toxicity is resolved. Children with upset tummies must therefore never be forced to eat! Their bodies need time to digest or expel the toxins before they become ready for any further nutritional input. Most of the common diseases of childhood represent pollution-control operations on the part of Nature to prevent the body from becoming laden with poisons. When these diseases are suppressed instead of being allowed to run their course, the ama remains behind, working its way deeper into the tissues where it can cause more complicated imbalances. Many—perhaps most—allergies and food sensitivities originate in a system that is filled with ama, and these allergies can go on to cause, or at least to reinforce, other potentially graver illnesses. For example, 95 percent of children who have allergies to nuts also have asthma, eczema, or hay fever.

Babies and Young Children

Ama is the cause of most disease, and the less you allow to collect in your child's body, the better her health will be, lifelong. The road to good health begins before conception, of course, and continues through gestation and delivery, but the days and weeks immediately following birth also offer splendid opportunities for training a child's physiology, metabolism, and psyche to prefer to function healthily.

Massage

The most beneficial habits should naturally be created first, which is why Ayurveda so passionately advocates massage for everyone, and particularly for infants. New mothers need regular massage, as do new babies. Babies in India are massaged for up to a year after they are born, and most traditions of mother and child care insist that, whatever the circumstances, both must be massaged for at least 40 days after delivery.

Baby massage stimulates the growing immune and nervous systems, and provides critical emotional nourishment. Some modern research suggests that premature infants who receive regular massage gain more weight and thrive more efficiently than do their peers who are not massaged. Infants who are not regularly cuddled and fondled can and do die; as late as 1920, the death rate for infants in orphanages in the United States was almost 100 percent. These orphanages, in which absolutely no bodily contact was provided to the babies, practiced the theories of men like Luther Emmett Holt, Sr. and J. B. Watson (the founder of behavioral psychology), who advised mothers to adopt fixed feeding schedules, a minimum of fondling, and strictness with toilet training.

Babies in India were once kept sequestered with their mothers for the first two weeks after birth, that they might have intimate contact with her all day and all night long during that critical fortnight. Even today, in most parts of India babies are kept indoors for their first 40 days of life. During this time they particularly require peace and quiet, for their tiny nervous systems are adjusting to the drastic shift from a quiet, fluid-filled existence to an air-filled world of intense sensory stimuli. Any "joint" aggravates vata, and there is particular danger that the transition from womb to room will create a potentially long-lasting vata-aggravation in the newborn. It is best during this period to keep the baby in an environment in which the lights and sounds are low and there are no intense odors (even ones you think are pleasant). Only a few of the baby's close relatives or family friends should be allowed to visit. The more time the mother spends with her baby during these 40 days, the better.

Oil massage is food for the baby's skin and nerves. It strengthens the skin, improves its color and texture, and makes it soft and smooth. The rhythmic movement relieves vata's erratic tendencies and alleviates stiffness, and the oil reduces vata's dry, light, and rough qualities. Sesame oil medicated with herbs is Ayurveda's traditional choice for a massage oil, but almond, olive, sunflower, or coconut oil can also be used, according to climate and availability. Never apply mineral oil or other inedible oils to your baby's skin. You can begin to massage your baby as soon as she is born, if you are careful not to touch her umbilical cord, or you can wait to begin until the cord falls off. Be sure that the room is warm and free of drafts, and that you massage her very gently. Speaking or singing sweetly to her as you stroke her body will please her immensely. Massage, which is a wonderful way to bond with a child, helps to calm any baby, even those of the sensitive, vata-provoked persuasion, and will improve her sleep. However, do not massage your baby when she is congested or otherwise out of balance.

Breastfeeding

A newborn baby's ideal food comes directly from her mother's breast. Science has shown that breastfeeding protects against such potentially grave diseases as gastroenteritis, respiratory illness, urinary tract infections, and necrotizing enterocolitis. Ayurveda teaches that mothers continue to transfer ojas to their children through their milk. Mothers in India used to breastfeed sweetness into their children for up to five years. Although the modern world has stolen such opportunities from most Indian urbanites, village and tribal women who do not live under time pressures continue to offer their own juices to their children long after they could get by on cooked food alone. Even today, in India's cities you can still see migrant construction workers along the roadside, hammer in one hand crushing rocks to pebbles, the other hand supporting a child avidly suckling at the breast.

In recent decades breastfeeding has been discouraged in many countries, and looked down upon in the West. Many Westerners still find it embarrassing—or scandalous—when they see a mother nursing her child in public. Despite this discouragement from society, try to breastfeed your baby for three months at the very least, and longer if possible. While you are nursing her, make sure that you replenish your own juices by eating adequate amounts of easy-to-digest food. Your body, which is working hard to make your baby healthy, deserves some pampering of its own.

If nursing your baby is not feasible, or if your milk doesn't come in well or flow well, you will have to try other milks. Be cautious with cow's milk, most of which has been highly processed by the time it reaches the consumer. Fresh goat's milk may be agreeable, or perhaps rice or oat milk. Soy milk is heavy for many babies. Breast milk is particularly handy, since whatever remedies the mother takes will flow, in milder form, into the baby when she nurses. Only a few herbs are given directly to an infant, such as dill water or fennel or mint tea, only a few drops at a time, on her tongue for colic.

Weaning

If you are able to breastfeed, you can start to wean your baby passively (by neglecting to offer her your breast) as soon as her milk teeth start to come in. You should start her on cooked food with gruel made from one grain—rice is especially good—to begin with. You can gradually add other grains, but in the beginning feed her only one grain at a meal. Gradually you can introduce strained vegetables, then strained fruits, then other foods into her diet, but always one new thing at a time. How she responds to specific foods may help you to understand her constitution better, and may enable you to notice promptly any sensitivities she might show to some of them. Respect her preferences: a healthy child will generally eat what her body knows it needs, not what you think it might require. The human body chooses its food according to the tastes it is missing.

Gradually introduce all six tastes into your child's diet, but delay introducing heavy, hard-to-manage foods like sesame, sticky dairy products such as yogurt, cheese, and ice cream, and concentrated high-protein and high-fat foods until her digestive tract is seasoned enough to withstand their effects (not less than a year). Pulses (legumes) are astringent, and green leafy vegetables both bitter and astringent; both thus promote vata. The best of the pungent digestive substances is ginger.

Constitution

What your child chooses to eat, and how it affects her, can tell you quite a lot about her constitution. You may have developed some suspicions even before her birth, of course, from dreams, feelings, or cravings, or from your experiences. Extremely active fetuses (vata) often become unusually anxious (vata) children, for instance. Still, you will learn much more about her after the birth. Since each child's constitution is fixed at the moment of conception, each newborn already has certain physical and mental "reaction prints" whose influence will grow progressively as she ages. It is no easy task to determine the constitution of a newborn baby, which means that it is better not to try to reach some immediate conclusion. Observe, and keep observing, and patterns will soon become evident.

Vata

Babies who are vata predominant are often more sensitive than the other types, in every way. They may startle easily, and may seem needlessly apprehensive. They often sleep less, or wake more often, and may cry suddenly and then stop just as suddenly for no apparent reason. Noise and cold may bother them. They often have irregular bowel movements, which may be hard and difficult to pass. They may pass a great deal of gas, and they may also tend to be colicky.

Pitta

Pitta-predominant babies rarely take no for an answer. When they want something they want it NOW, and may bellow until they get it, particularly if it is food. Sleep may not interest them much. They usually enjoy eating and digest well, although they may be prone to loose stools when they overeat or are over-stimulated. Their skin, which is often sensitive to the sun, may be as irritable as their temperament.

Kapha

Babies in whom kapha is in the ascendant are often more placid and less sensitive than the other two types. They tend to have big bones, and may put on weight easily. They also tend to be more regular in their eating, sleeping, and bowel habits, and are more likely to sleep through the night than their compatriots from the other doshas.

Remember, though, that few people are uni-doshic in constitution, and your baby is likely to have one primary dosha and one that, although secondary, will still occasionally rise up to throw its weight around. Also, whatever your baby's personal constitution may be, children are basically kapha predominant because childhood is the kapha season of life. This is why they grow easily, sleep a lot, rebound quickly from disease or injury, and are often exquisitely emotionally sensitive.

Feeding

While as a mother your job is to set an example for your children in everything you do, this is especially true in the context of food. Although this may eat away at your own free time, it is the best investment that you can make in their (and possibly your) future. It is easy to fill up a belly temporarily in a fast-food restaurant, but that fast food (which, like anything fast, is vata-provoking) will probably leave both mind and soul unsatisfied. From the very beginning, your children need to experience practical proof of how well a small amount of food, lovingly presented, can satisfy you—body, mind, and spirit.

Some people never learn to cook, but there is every reason to entice your sons and daughters into the kitchen to encourage them to try. As you whip, purée, stir-fry, and sauté a variety of foods, your offspring will soak up details about healthy eating that few of them would sit still long enough to listen to. One of the first things they will need to know, no doubt, is what sorts of food will promote health and which will not. But selecting what you will eat is only part of eating. The other, often more important part, is knowing how to eat. At a minimum, your children need to learn the basic principles of healthy eating.

Sweets

Despite what anyone may tell you, nothing in life is guaranteed, and it is better to get used to this idea as soon as you become pregnant. No matter how perfect an example you set for your children, or how excellent an environment you create for them, they are their own persons, and as they develop they will inevitably go their own ways.

Children love the sweet taste, which they need to feed their growing bodies. It is as easy for them to become addicted to "empty" sweets like chocolate as it may be difficult for you to discourage them from their consumption. There is no doubt that in the average child sugary treats imbalance the blood sugar and increase adrenalin levels, producing the exact opposite of the calm satisfaction that wholesome sweet food should produce. But you cannot legislate your child's life. As a parent, all you can do is provide her with good food, and try to develop in her from an early age a taste for sweets that have good effects on the body. Put healthy sweets in front of her—carrots, fresh fruits, dates, figs, granola—and then stand back and hope for the best.

Puberty and Menarche

Some ama-based conditions, such as acne and mood swings, may not become evident until they are triggered by the hormonal changes of puberty. Adolescence is the transition between childhood and adulthood—it is the "joint" at which these two very different stages of life meet. Since childhood is ruled by kapha, adulthood by pitta, and "joints" by vata, there is ample opportunity for all three doshas to go out of alignment during the teenage years.

This is particularly true now that modern life is altering the timing of the moment when some individuals become physiologically capable of sexual reproduction. When influenced by the external conditions in which they find themselves, many mammals can change the age at which they reach puberty, and members of the human species who live in the temperate regions of the industrialized world have been reaching puberty earlier in recent years. Partly, at least, this has to do with light, for, like other animals, humans seem to have circa-annual (about a year) cycles which involve changes in blood chemistry, hormone secretion, brain activity, and appetite. These cycles are based on day-to-day changes in the length of daylight and darkness. In the past, girls in the tropics tended to reach puberty earlier than did girls in higher latitudes, presumably because they were exposed more consistently to bright light than were their peers elsewhere. Now, however, high-intensity artificial lighting at home, at school, and in the shopping mall seem to be replicating the influence of the tropical sun, and stimulating the reproductive systems of non-tropical girls so that they resemble those of their more equatorial cousins.

But light is probably not the only factor involved here. Some researchers have proposed that a home filled with parental strife, or one where the father is absent because of divorce or abandonment, induces the girls who are raised within it to reach puberty at an earlier age. They argue that species which rely on stable environments (like the elephant) tend to have larger bodies, live longer, have longer gestations and reach puberty later than do opportunistic species (like desert plants, or animals that live near seasonal waterholes), who live boom-and-bust existences. Opportunistic species are gamblers; they have smaller bodies and are shorter-lived. Following this line of reasoning, girls abandoned by their fathers tend to grow up more like opportunistic species, and so reach puberty sooner.

Even if this hypothesis of parental stress is true, it cannot be the only explanation, for young athletes and anorexics are also stressed, and they tend to have later puberties than their calmer peers. Other influences surely contribute, including the many estrogen-like chemicals that appear everywhere in the modern environment; heightened exposure to microwaves, ultraviolet light, and other forms of radiation; and the stress of loud noise and subsonic vibrations. Each girl will respond differently to these many determinants, according to her own personal proclivities, but all these factors will increase vata. The result is a massive epidemic of aggravated vata, which is itself a major cause of menstrual dysfunction.

These physical disturbances are yet further aggravated by modern society, which is working hard to change the nature of adolescence itself. Adolescence is the time when a young woman becomes possessed by the shakti—the power of creation. Like all other energies, creativity must be properly harnessed in order to be useful; left unchanneled, it can destroy. Electricity can light your home or electrocute you; fire can cook your food or cremate you; wind can turn a windmill or blow it over. Any wave can hold you up or suck you under, depending on how you position yourself on top of it. Similarly, the creative wave that is youth must be harnessed carefully if it is to prove a productive time of life rather than a decade of strife.

The Three Pillars

The first thing to remember when considering how to have a trouble-free (or at least hassle-reduced) adolescence is that three of life's activities are most in need of quantity control. The *Charaka Samhita* calls them life's main supports, or its "three pillars": sleep, eating, and sexual activity.

Sleep

Sleep allows the mind to digest, via dreams. Children dream more than adults, and fetuses seem to dream all the time (Ayurveda suggests that this is because they are reliving the experiences of previous existences in preparation for their next one). Insufficient sleep makes the mind and body duller and less adaptable, and aggravates vata yet further.

Youngsters are unusual in that until their mid-twenties they seem to have a circadian rhythm that is closer to twenty-six hours than to the twenty-five hours which is the norm for adults. Also, in the absence of specific light cues (which they do not get if they spend most of their time skulking around indoors) their times for sleeping and waking get pushed ahead, making them sleep and wake later. Since teenagers usually need nine to eleven hours of sleep each day, and during the school week will often try to get by on seven or eight hours, they create for themselves a sizeable sleep debt by the weekend. They try to pay off this debt by sleeping later then, but waking at noon resets their internal clocks to make them sleepy again only at 4 A.M. If you are a teenager, you can escape from this plight by maintaining a more constant sleep-wake schedule. Get out of bed on weekends no later than an hour after your normal rising time (you can always take an afternoon nap if you need one), and go outside as soon as you rise in order to expose yourself to some daylight. Your body will thank you for it!

Food

A well-rested body will be far more enthusiastic about eating and digesting than an annoyed, sleep-deprived one. We have already mentioned how important food is to health, and if you make a point of eating healthily most of the time, your body will probably have little difficulty in coping with the occasional excess. The food chart in appendix 1 can help you make dietary choices, but remember that each individual's requirements are unique, and are never entirely predictable. Eating food that pacifies your predominant dosha is usually best, but when you are going through upheaval, a vata-calming diet is likely to benefit almost anyone.

Eating disorders

Most common childhood diseases are communicable, traded from family to family. Children are frequently more open than adults to new things, and some of these will unfortunately make them sick. One of the most malignant of the several epidemics that is surging through the West today is that of dysmorpho-phobia, or "fear of having a misshapen body." Repeated exposure from a young age to our current ideal of beauty—thin, leggy, nearly hipless—teaches girls and young women (and also their mothers) to evaluate their worth in terms of their appearance. One recent survey suggested that more than 80 percent of nine-year-olds in California have already been on a diet, while a 1996 national survey of 2,379 girls aged nine and ten showed that 40 percent had tried to lose weight. Among this group were girls who were overweight, normal in weight, even underweight. Those most likely to try to lose weight were those who were either overweight or whose mothers told them that they were overweight. (In general, black girls were satisfied with a less thin version of "thin" than were white girls.)

If the situation is bad at these ages, it intensifies exponentially as puberty dawns, breasts begin to bud, and hips begin to reveal themselves. Seventy percent of teenage girls in the United Sates diet, and some of the girls and young women who crave to become "ideal women" starve themselves in that direction. Others exercise fanatically, which causes many female athletes to reach puberty later than their peers, or to stop menstruating for months or years at a time. Some athletes go so far overboard that they develop osteoporosis at a young age; this happens when they become so over-conditioned that their total body fat falls below the minimum level that the body needs in order to produce its hormones. Taken to its extremes, dieting can lead to anorexia and bulimia, which are at epidemic levels: about 20 percent of college women in the United States have eating disorders. Anorexia, bulimia, and binge-eating currently affect seven million women in the U.S., although they are no longer exclusively "female" diseases. Now one million young men are affected too; a recent study among Cornell University football players showed that 40 percent of them had dysfunctional eating patterns, and 10 percent outright eating disorders.

Sex

Football players and other athletes commonly excuse their eating behavior on the grounds of "having to make the weight" to get or stay on the team, but this is only one side of the story. The other side is, for many people, a belief that thinness equals sexual attractiveness. Adolescence is the time when sexual individuality begins to crystallize, and there are few teenagers who don't want to look good for someone. This realm of life has come particularly strongly into focus in the latter half of the twentieth century, when to choose to be sexually inactive has come to be regarded as positively unhealthy.

Sex is more open and readily available in our society than ever before, but very few people are really sexually satisfied. In fact, the more titillated people become, the more frustrated they seem to be. This frustration usually begins in teenhood, as peer pressure to "perform" forces girls and boys into sexually charged situations well before they are ready to face them, either emotionally or physically.

Simply because you have passed the age of puberty and are physiologically ready to reproduce does not mean that the sexual experience will be effortlessly satisfying for you, any more than fruit is ready to eat the moment it appears on the tree. Flavor appears in fruit only after it has ripened and is ready to fall; if you pick it early, or apply chemicals to it to speed its maturation, you will lose the chance to enjoy the juices that the natural ripening process will engender within it. A healthy, satisfying, sexual relationship requires time and energy to develop, and today very few people give sex enough of either. Instead, what usually happens is that before the energy even gets a chance to accumulate it becomes dissipated. Even before the fruit has had the opportunity to ripen it is shaken loose from the tree, and told to mature on its own and to go out and locate its own nourishment.

All teenagers would do well to minimize their sexual play until their body-mind-spirit complexes are fully developed. But it is unreasonable to expect that the young will simply sit back and refrain from sexual activity on their own. Unless they are shown how to refine and accumulate, safely and practically, the flood of creativity that is within them, its current will continue to drive them crazy. This is why this first stage of life, from birth until the end of physical growth, was in India traditionally set aside for physical, mental, and spiritual development, and during this period students were expected to be sexually continent, in order to allow the energy which was needed for satisfying life experiences to accumulate. However, they were not left to their own devices, as so many youngsters are today; rather, their mentors taught them in detail how to cultivate and channel their energies, and how to direct them toward the accomplishment of their aims.

Rejuvenation

Today few young girls have mentors, and many succumb to the lure of some excess, if not sexual then in some other realm: athletics, intoxicants, gangs, shopping. One can become addicted to anything, and becoming conditioned to something harmful at an early age risks setting yourself up for an addiction that may dog you for the rest of your life.

Some addictions are quite unforgiving, but most produce damage that can be repaired, particularly if you begin reconstruction while you are still young. The younger you are when you embark on the journey toward good health, the easier it will be to attain your goal, but you can get there whenever you set sail. The worst approach to unhealthy behavior is to resign yourself to it, telling yourself that you are too weak or helpless to change, or that the damage has already been done. Have faith in your body, which possesses an amazing capacity to regenerate its parts. (So amazing, in fact, that in the same way that certain species can actually regrow limbs that have been severed, a human fingertip that is accidentally chopped off will regrow, within three months, as long as the child that owns it is less than eleven years old.) Most people have sufficient vitality to endure years of riotous living before major damage is done, but the sum of even two decades' worth of burgers and chips is likely to require several months of remedial eating at the very least to allow your organism to scrub away its accumulated ama and rejuvenate itself.

Rejuvenation (*rasayana* in Sanskrit) is intended to return your body-mind-spirit complex to an earlier state of natural integration, to prevent diseases that are preventable, and to minimize those which cannot be avoided. The *Charaka Samhita* speaks of two types of rasayana: with substances and without. Teenagers can benefit from many sorts of rejuvenative substances. For example, one in seven adolescent girls in the United States has low iron, mainly because of blood loss through menses. Diets supplemented with iron can enhance their physical vitality, and can even improve some aspects of their cognitive functioning. Unfortunately, most of the commercial iron supplements available, which are meant to be absorbed directly by the body, are not well tolerated by the digestive tract. Ayurveda, which seeks instead substances that can be absorbed indirectly and more slowly, converts the minerals and metals it uses therapeutically into oxides by means of combining them with herbs and incinerating them repeatedly. This process improves a mineral's availability to the body by, among other things, reducing its particle size and loading it with a subtle form of oxygen. Ayurvedically prepared iron *(loha bhasma)* is often rejuvenative for anemic women, particularly those whose diets have been impoverished in other nutrients as well. In such cases, Ayurvedic supplements like *chyvanaprasha* (see page 88) can offer preventive care.

SKIN-CARE ROUTINE

My mentor proposed the following daily skin-care regimen for a pimple-afflicted face:

Cut a slice from a fresh lime and scrub the skin gently with it for a few seconds, before thoroughly washing off the juice with warm (not hot) water. Then take a palmful of dry oats (the kind you might cook for your breakfast), add enough water to them to make a paste, and scrub the skin thoroughly. Leave the oat paste on until it dries, then wash it off with very warm water. Allow the skin to breathe for some time before you apply anything else (such as cosmetics) to it.

Rejuvenating the Skin

The tissue which most often needs rejuvenating in a young woman is her skin. The transition that is adolescence stirs up any ama that has been accumulating in the system for the past few years or so, and if the organs of excretion are not prepared to handle that extra burden, the toxins will try to exit through the skin. Acne is a teen-year affliction that can often be helped by diet, exercise, and internal use of preparations like triphala and aloe vera, but external attention is also welcome.

Any cosmetics that you do wear should be as mild and unreactive as possible, so as to avoid aggravating the pitta that is already fired up in blemish-prone skin. Herbal-based facial scrubs and lotions may also be helpful, particularly if you know what effect their ingredients will have on your doshas. Some Ayurvedic preparations are specially formulated with rejuvenative herbs to encourage the skin to return to a balanced state.

Rejuvenative herbal creams can also revitalize the skin of your body, particularly when they are supplemented with regular massage. Ideally, you began receiving massage shortly after you were born; if not, now is a good time to begin! You should choose a massage oil carefully, for some of its ingredients are likely to be absorbed into your system through your skin. This is why preparations which contain mineral oil (a petroleum-based product) are usually inappropriate for regular use on your body.

Substance-free Rejuvenation

This is how the process of substance-free rejuvenation is described by the famous Ayurvedic text *Ashtanga Hridaya:*

> *Those who speak the truth, who never become angry,*
> *who lead a spiritually pure life and are always serene are*
> *considered to be rejuvenated daily.*

Modern scientists are confirming a truth long known and practiced by yogis, that there are two ways in which life can be extended: by eating the minimum amount of food to preserve your life, and by lowering your body temperature. But lowering your mental temperature is also essential. All passion is hot, and heat destroys ojas. A fiery temperament decreases your chances of extended survival; a cool head promotes longevity.

Daily rejuvenation is facilitated by purifying your body of residual doshas and ama, and by resisting the temptation to consume intoxicants (especially alcohol) and other substances that promote dosha aggravation and ama production. Meditation and prayer are also essential elements in the daily rejuvenating routine, because they help you to eliminate from your life the mental ama that conflicts and negative emotions create. The calmer you become, the more harmonious will be the energy you create, or draw to you.

You should complement this regular cleansing of physical and psychic sludge by focusing on rebuilding your organism. The best way to do this is to imbibe, with proper digestion and assimilation, foods and ideas of the sweet taste. Sweetness should become a part of your life: your speech should promote harmony, your manner should be gently compassionate, your life calmly routine, and your awareness simple and respectful of life and Nature.

This whole process may seem a tall order, but try to comply as best you can. The more strictly that you follow this regimen, the better it will work for you. The recuperative powers of the young are such that teenagers and young adults who can make even minimal attempts to comply with this prescription will usually benefit from it.

Four

WOMANHOOD

THE PITTA AGE

If you were fortunate enough to learn healthy ways of living as a child, you probably entered your adult life trusting the universe's inherent munificence, confident that you would at least be able to cope with whatever life served up to you. If you did not, now is a good time to learn! Even if you were not conceived, or did not grow up, in an optimal way, there is still time for you to train yourself, or to allow someone to train you, to live in that healthy space with those healthy flows.

As long as there is life, there is the chance to learn to trust it. And learning to trust will be an easier task for you if you are able to re-enter, even briefly, the attitude of innocence and wonder that you enjoyed when you were a little girl. This does not necessarily mean that you should try to pamper your "inner child"—particularly if your inner child happens to be a petulant or bossy little thing. If, however, she is cheerful and happy-go-lucky, then she may well act as a reminder to you of what life can be; otherwise, you and she may simply find yourselves engaging in some very self-indulgent and potentially destructive interactions.

It may not be easy to find the time and space to realign your flow when you are living through the pitta time in your life. Pitta

REMEMBER LIFE'S BASIC PRINCIPLES

- Life is relationship.

- The most important of all relationships is the one a woman has with herself.

- A living human being is a body-mind-spirit complex.

- Matter develops from consciousness, and an organism's consciousness continually seeks to express itself through the matter that makes up its body-mind.

- All flows in all parts of an organism interact with and influence one another; the flow of influence is predominantly from subtler to denser.

likes to manage, and the average adult woman today seems to spend all her time doing nothing but that. Partner and children, parents, work, finances—all tug at her, demanding her attention. In such a situation it is very easy for her attention to fragment, and when that happens her prana fragments, which causes her vata to lose its cohesion. Erratic vata incites pitta, kapha, the tissues, and the wastes to go out of balance, and if nothing is done to redress the situation a disease will result—possibly some sort of metabolic disorder, which is characteristic of pitta.

Fragmentation happens not only when your life seems to be falling apart completely; it can also occur more insidiously. Things might be going so well in one of life's arenas (your job, for instance) that it may take a major imbalance to make you notice that another area (like your emotional life) has fallen into disarray. For whatever reason, women seem somehow to be more afflicted by today's hectic lifestyle than are men, and the results can be tragic. Seven out of every ten prescriptions for psychoactive medicines go to women, and the suicide rate for female physicians and psychologists is three times higher than that for their male counterparts.

Finding the Center

What is the answer? Reconnect with the center of life. Unless the life you create for yourself is flowing along in harmony with Nature's flow, you will find yourself slogging through existential fear and despair as the firm ground beneath your feetslips away. If that should be happening to you, here are a few suggestions for gaining back some traction.

Look back. Remember a moment from your earlier life when you felt happy, healthy, safe, and relaxed. Maybe it was during your childhood or your adolescence, maybe during early adulthood. Whenever it was, return yourself completely to that moment, and let the feelings you had then flood you until you are swimming in them. Then, floating in that feeling, return your conscious mind to the present time and try to overlay your current condition with those pleasing feelings.

Look forward. Consider ways in which you can simplify your life. If you don't even have time to think, ferret out some time for yourself (if necessary, without letting anyone else know what you are doing) and do something with it that makes you feel really nurtured—even if that something is nothing more than taking a catnap. Once you are feeling rested and renewed, review your priorities carefully. You are sure to find something that you can eliminate, or postpone, or reduce, and when you do, you will be at least that much less fragmented.

Look around. Find a mentor, a wise and trusted counselor. She need not be older than you, or even necessarily a woman, but it should be someone who is interested in you and who has a better perspective than you do on what is going on in your life. She may have practical hints on how to restructure, revitalize, and renew yourself, or she may simply be a wise woman who nourishes you with her presence alone. Ayurveda strongly counsels every woman to spend all her extra time with benevolent, compassionate wise ones.

Look within. Mother Nature lives within all of us, all of the time. Once you have learned to contact her, you will never feel lonely again. That moment from your past when you felt integrated and whole was a moment when her hand was on your shoulder. The inspiration you receive when you take time for yourself to reflect is engendered by her. The advice your mentor gives you comes from Mother Nature, speaking through the mentor's mouth. Wherever you are, you can always put yourself into Nature's presence, if you can learn where to find her.

Looking Within

It is no doubt difficult to know where or how to locate Mother Nature when you feel overwhelmed by darkness, but if you reach out to her, she will extend her hand to you. One way to reach out is to try to identify within yourself the gifts she gives us. These are many, but from the point of view of physical health the most important are prana, tejas, and ojas. Here is one method:

1. **Sit with your back comfortably straight and your body at rest.** Close your eyes and start to focus on your breath. As you breathe out, allow all your physical, mental, and emotional tightness and anxiety to flow out with your breath. As you breathe in, breathe in the gentle golden light of the rising sun and let it permeate every part of you. If any thoughts arise to interrupt your reverie, gently sweep them from your field of awareness (if they are important, they will return).

2. **Now start to follow the breath as it enters your body-mind.** Let your awareness move with your breath, and see where that awareness takes you. In the beginning it may not take you very far, which is normal. Keep trying, and before too long you will find yourself becoming able to distinguish between the current of

your breath and the current of the energy that your breath brings into you. That energy is prana. As you follow the prana through your organism you will find it moving smoothly in some places and becoming obstructed in others. As you become practiced at this, you will learn to redirect prana to those areas within you that most need it by using nothing more than the force of your breathing and your awareness. (Vata people: make sure you do not rev up your nervous energy with this practice!)

3. **Once you are able to follow your prana, follow it down into your cells.** One of prana's jobs is to inflame the body's tejas. If prana is the breath of life, tejas is the flame of life, the healthy fire that transforms all the physical, energetic, emotional, mental, and spiritual things that we consume into parts of ourselves. Like prana, tejas exists in each cell, and if you can follow the prana as it penetrates your body deeper and deeper, down to the level of your cells, you can use it to breathe life into this fire. Again, you will find as you examine your body-mind-spirit that in some areas of life your fire is cooking along quite well and in others it is not. Maybe it has burned down to embers in one location, or is pouring out thick black smoke as it tries to ignite some wet fuel somewhere else. Gently rebuild those of your fires that have died down, and as you do you will soon be able to sense a glow of health arising within you as your reinvigorated cells radiate subtle warmth into your consciousness. (Pitta people: do not permit this practice to make you hotheaded!)

4. **As soon as your tejas is well kindled you can use it to help build up ojas.** Envision a dish of warm, liquid ghee (clarified butter), and coat your body thinly with it (this should feel good in and of itself). Now, carefully layer a film of pure honey on top of the ghee. As the flame of your tejas ignites these substances, instead of burning, they will transform themselves into a thick band of golden-yellow light that covers your whole body and radiates out into space. This ghee-honey cushion is similar in

color and consistency to ojas, the semi-physical material that produces your aura and grants your immunity. The stronger your ojas, the better-integrated you will be, and feel yourself to be. (Kapha people: do not let this practice clog you up or make you complacent!)

5. **Remain in this state of balance as long as you like (or can).** Then, gradually open your eyes. Retaining at least the flavor of these three awarenesses in your conscious awareness, return to the process of going about your business.

The varieties of meditation are innumerable, and if this type does nothing for you, then take up another one, or begin to pray regularly. But do something to initiate the process of aligning yourself with the one thing that is truly important in the universe: your relationship with Reality, by whichever name you prefer to call it (God, Mother Nature, the Goddess, the Great Spirit). You can commune with Reality on the beach of a tropical island within yourself no matter where you are, if that image becomes real for you. Ayurveda asks you to remember your Creator, that you may allow the Creator's pulse of health to enter into you and remind you what health feels and looks and tastes like.

Routine: The Five Vatas

However you choose to meditate, you are likely to find greater success at readjusting the flow of your thoughts after you have invested some time and energy in balancing your body and your doshas. You can begin by developing a daily routine, even a minimalist one, to begin encouraging healthy cycles in your prana and vata. Arising before dawn is a handy way to enter the new diurnal cycle awake and alert, and it also allows you to use the increased force of vata during that part of the day to encourage your body to eliminate its wastes. Urine and feces are expelled from the body by apana, which is one of vata's five subdoshas. Although there is actually only one force of vata in the body, this one force flows in different directions in different parts of the body. (Pitta and kapha have subdoshas as well, but in the context of flow, vata's subdoshas deserve more attention.)

Vata's five subdoshas divide the body into five different spheres of influence:

1. **Prana vata,** the "forward-moving air," rules the functions of the heart, lungs, and esophagus. Its field of activity extends from the diaphragm to the throat, and it is in charge of taking things like food, water, and air into the system. All five vatas are derived from prana, the life force, but since prana vata is so involved with the intake of the life force, it received its parent's name.

2. **Udana vata,** the "upward-moving air," whose field extends from the throat to the top of the head, controls self-expression: speech, endeavor, enthusiasm, memory, vitality, complexion, and the like.

3. **Samana vata,** the "equalizing air," extends from the diaphragm to the navel. It supervises digestion and assimilation, and helps keep prana and apana in balance.

4. **Vyana vata,** the "pervasive air," permeates the entire body from its seat in the heart. Vyana distributes nourishment through the system and regulates such activities as circulation of the blood and lymph, locomotion, and perspiration.

5. **Apana vata,** the "downward-moving air," operates from the navel to the anus. It is responsible for expelling things from the body: urine, feces, gas, semen, menstrual blood, and the fetus (at the time of delivery).

Elimination

Because no healthy flow is possible when the channels of the body and mind are clogged with wastes, the free and fearless movement of apana is essential to everyone's health. It is for this reason that Ayurvedic teachers have for centuries reinforced in their students the importance of healthy elimination.

It is usually not too difficult to train your colon to empty itself each morning, and when you do you should inspect the wastes therefrom (at least cursorily). Healthy urine is clear and light-colored; healthy feces are light brown with the consistency of a ripe banana. Neither has much odor. Remember that turbid, foul-smelling urine and sticky feces that are offensive in odor and contain pieces of undigested food signal the presence of ama (toxins due to improperly digested food). So does a thick coating on your tongue, rank breath, and fetid sweat.

Ama promotes disease in many ways: it obstructs the free movement of vata and prana, weakens the digestive fire while aggravating pitta, and perverts the functioning of ojas and kapha. Ama also acts as food for physical, mental, and emotional parasites. When signs of ama like those listed above appear, especially when they are accompanied by some or all of the symptoms listed below, acute accumulation of ama may have occurred in your system.

In such situations it is wise to fast for the day, or at least to skip a meal. This will give your body the time and space to digest the toxins undisturbed.

Symptoms of Accumulated Ama

- Obstruction to major channels of flow.

- Lethargy, accompanied by a feeling of heaviness in the limbs and/or mind.

- Fatigue and/or loss of strength without exertion.

- Nausea and/or indigestion.

- Retention of wastes, especially inhibition of sweating.

- Experiencing food as tasteless, or, for common foods, as having unusual tastes.

Exercise

A good time to take gentle exercise is soon after your digestive tract has rid itself of its wastes. Exercise is food for those people whose muscle mass it helps increase, it is medicine for the obese, and poison for those who become addicted to it. Exercise addiction can develop in those who use it for tension release, in those who crave the endorphin thrills it delivers, or in those who rely on it to enhance their self-image. Excessive exercise can cause physical injury, and may actually shorten your lifespan. It can also create severe and lasting vata imbalances. Only kapha-type people really need a vigorous and long daily workout; everyone else, especially vata types, should be more moderate. In fact, over-exercising can be positively dangerous to vata types. As many as one in every four people who perform four hours or more a week of high-impact aerobics develops vertigo, dizziness, loss of balance, tinnitus, or even hearing loss, all of which are vata-type conditions. Take it easy!

It is rarely appropriate to expend more than half your available energy on exercise at any one time if you are exercising for the benefit of your health. If, for example, you become exhausted after running for an hour, you ought not to run for more than half an hour at a time until you build up your stamina. Generally, you can tell that you have exercised enough to strengthen your circulatory system when sweat appears on your forehead. Strenuous exercise is also contraindicated in cases of severe indigestion, in advanced vata diseases such as chronic respiratory complaints, in intense pitta conditions like blood disorders and severe inflammations, and for the very young and very old.

Whatever sort of strenuous exercise you may choose to pursue, you should supplement it with some type of "energy work" like hatha yoga, tai chi or qi gong. Energy work encourages all five of vata's subdoshas to remain within their own respective spheres, co-operating efficiently with one another. Properly practiced, such exercise will promote the free flow of prana in your organism, it will stimulate the tejas within your cells, and encourage the development of better immunity and resilience by enhancing your production of ojas.

A little self-massage with oil is a good way to round off your exercise, and after a quick shower or bath to wash away any wastes discharged through the skin, you can eliminate some of your mental wastes by meditation. If meditation doesn't seem to work for you, at least take a few moments each morning to marvel over the miracle of existence, over the day that is about to begin, and all its untapped potential. Allow this miracle to instill a deep-felt reverence for all life in the core of your being, and request Nature to maintain and amplify your own harmony during the day, so that you will interact harmoniously with everyone and everything you encounter, and your own harmony will increase.

Even if you do nothing else, the act of involving yourself in a daily routine enables your organism to make changes that can exert positive effects on your health, by reducing ama and promoting the free movement of the five vatas. Unless you have lived a life of purity and balance from your very conception, you are bound to have some ama stored somewhere in your body, and this has to emerge eventually and then be expelled from the body. It will appear in its own good time; but you can create conditions that will encourage such purification to occur, while discouraging any more ama from forming.

Imbalance: Prajnaparadha

Unless you are a saint, you will go out of balance and become sick from time to time. Occasional sickness is inevitable for a mortal; continuously perfect health does not exist on our planet. Every body-mind-spirit has some weak point, somewhere, that serves as the theater in which the doshas act out their drama. Every individual has some ego-calcification that tempts her into *prajnaparadha* from time to time.

Prajnaparadha—literally, "an offense against wisdom"—happens whenever one part of you insists on an action that is detrimental to the rest of you. It happens when you know deep inside that something is not right for your body-mind-spirit, but you obstinately go ahead and do it anyway, ignoring Nature's warnings. Any part of you can perform prajnaparadha, from the cancerous cell that rebels against the organism's wisdom, to the mind that insists on its idiosyncratic version of reality. Ayurvedists who survey today's world find prajnaparadha everywhere they look, and are not surprised to discover gargantuan imbalances emerging as rampant disease.

My mentor, the Aghori Vimalananda, was very big on the real reality. "It is always better to live with reality," he would say, "because otherwise, without fail, reality will come to live with you." While you are a child you live in a world of seemingly unlimited possibilities. As you become an adult, limitations set in, and you learn that you have to live within your limits if you want to enjoy unimpeded flow. Life without limits perverts your reality; it sours your sweetness, or turns it bitter. Sickness is "reality coming to live with you," which is why it is all right to be sick. Sickness is Nature's tap on your shoulder, her reminder to you that you have strayed from the path. When you open yourself to her again, and allow her to work within you, she will reawaken your body's innate healing abilities to set things right. Until you return to that path, Nature will go on reminding you, for as long as it takes—or until your viability as a body-mind-spirit complex expires. How well your natural healing mechanisms will work in any specific instance depends mainly on two things: how carefully you follow the appropriate regimen (without being stiff and humorless about it), and how much vitality your system retains. After all, everyone has to die of something.

When you are sick, you should ask yourself practical questions, such as how to change your ways so that your disease will disappear. Do not, however, fall into the trap of trying to figure out what you did to bring this on yourself. However well meaning are the New Age types who offer this fundamentalist sort of advice, there is little to be gained by getting stuck on some simplistic cause-effect relationship when you are trying to extricate yourself from the jaws of a disease. You will do better to focus on regaining your health instead of trying to conduct an autopsy on how you went wrong.

Because it is always best to detect and correct imbalances while they are still incubating, it is useful to learn about your own physical, energetic, mental, and emotional "blind spots" and then try to keep a regular eye on them. You should try to pay attention to yourself when you are feeling fine, so that you will quickly take notice when you are not feeling right. The earlier you can detect that something is wrong with you, even if it is not detectable on any of the standard diagnostic tests, the sooner you can treat yourself and prevent the disease from needing to manifest itself fully. This also applies, of course, to everyone you are parenting. It is good to keep a watch on your children, by such means as their pulses, voices, or food habits, and try to nip any problems in the bud.

You will find it easier to recognize blind spots if you can also identify strengths. Perhaps the most striking of the many differences between Ayurveda and Western medicine is that while the latter focuses on disease to the extent that it defines health as its absence, Ayurveda focuses on health. Ayurvedic diagnosis, therefore, begins with what is right with you: how well nourished, toned, and "excellent" your tissues are, and how effectively your channels flow.

Excellences

Ayurveda paints a picture of those people in whom all factors of bodily health are excellent and in perfect tone that shows them enjoying firm, well-knit bodies. They have smooth, soft, lustrous skin, shining eyes, and resonant, mellow, strong voices. They walk with a firm tread. Ojas, the essence of immune power, creates a powerfully protective and attractive aura around them. They are strong but gentle, self-confident in their enterprises, and able to bear troubles cheerfully. They busy themselves happily with worthy pursuits and enjoy all pleasures in appropriate fashion. Often such people become powerful and wealthy, and are honored by their neighbors. Both they and their offspring are slow to age or to be attacked by disease, and live long. Such people are endowed with what the Ayurvedic texts call "joyful circumstances" as the recipients of that marvellous blessing known as good health, and the metabolic joy that their cells feel overflows into their outer environment, where it encourages health to flourish. To live in the aura of such people can improve your own health, happiness, and peace of mind. Conversely, living around imbalanced individuals may perturb you in the same way that a polluted habitat pollutes its inhabitants.

Such excellence of mind includes strong memory, devotion, gratitude, wisdom, purity, energy, skill, courage, freedom from sorrow, deep intelligence, and solid character. Mental excellence is in many ways superior to the bodily kind, because the strong-minded busy themselves with worthy pursuits even when their bodies lack perfect health.

- Strong-minded people are affected minimally by severe ailments even if they are weak in body.

- Those whose minds are moderately powerful seek consolation for their miseries from others, and console themselves by comparing themselves to others.

- Weak-minded people cannot be calmed and recomposed either by themselves or by others. Even if they are strong in body, the weak-minded cannot tolerate even small ailments stoically, and they may become unhinged when shocked by fear, sorrow, temptation, delusion, or disgrace.

The stronger a person's mind, the more likely it is that he or she will be able to "digest" unpleasant experiences and emerge from them less vulnerable to future imbalance than before.

Excellences of body and mind are a good measure of a person's strength and vitality, for they provide good indications of life's momentum. It is easy to be deceived by a body's appearance unless you examine its excellences. According to the *Charaka Samhita*, major diseases can seem minor in people who have "richness of spirit, vitality and body," while minor diseases can seem major in a patient with "poverty" of those things. Robust people with big bodies are not necessarily strong, nor are emaciated people, nor are those with small bodies necessarily weak. In all aspects of life and living, size is less important than proportion. The extent to which your life will be filled with vitality, happiness, power, wealth, and other benefits often depends mainly on how well you can apportion your time and space to the tasks that your life has assigned you.

Less-than-Excellences

The last thing you would want to conclude after reading the paragraphs above is that you are so far from the ideal that there is no hope of ever getting there. There is every likelihood that you can get closer to that ideal than you are now. Your system likes having such an image of health to work toward, because it gives the organism something around which it can organize itself, just as the pearl organizes itself around a grain of sand.

Let us assume that you have improved your diet and habits—at least a little. Now you need to examine carefully your current state of health/ill-health, which is expressed by the dosha balance in your condition (vikriti). Part of your vikriti comes from the impact of your diet and habits on the dosha-aggravating tendencies of your constitution (prakriti), part from the consequences of the various seasons, and part from your personal strengths and weakness and your level of prajnaparadha. The rest derives from the influence on you of the animals, vegetables, minerals, radiations, and vibrations of the environment in which you live. Everything with which you relate influences you, for better or worse. It is no accident that people with pitta-kapha or kapha-pitta constitutions tend to "succeed at success" today more easily than do other constitutional types. They are the ones who can continue to resonate with prosperity even when they are exposed to the extremely fast, imbalanced, intense, vata-provoking modern world in which we now live.

The sum of the repercussions of all these influences produces your "state," your body-mind-spirit's personal pattern of flow relationships. Your state, which is the sum of your past and present, points the way toward your future, on all levels of your existence. When something or someone "gets you into a state," that state is who you are for the time you remain in it.

When you are in a state, the whole of your body-mind-spirit usually enters that state, although most states choose one level of existence on which to manifest most strongly. Imbalances that begin in one location can very well surface elsewhere, and balance that begins on one level can communicate itself to other levels. Furthermore, just as physical illness can be generated from disturbances of the mind or the prana, and mental disorders may arise from financial derangements, in the same way harmony of the mind or spirit or prana can prove infectious to every other consciousness in your organism.

Evaluating symptoms

Careful evaluation of your symptoms when you are feeling unwell can allow you to discern your immediate pattern of dosha involvement, or at the very least to determine which dosha most urgently requires correction. One useful general rule is:

There is no pain without vata, no inflammation without pitta, and no pus formation without kapha.

The greater the pain, the more vata is involved; the more fiery the inflammation, the angrier the pitta; the larger the volume of pus, the greater the kapha. Colic is a vata type of pain, sunburn and ulcer give pitta-type pain, and kapha pain is that of a stuffed-up nose. A cough which produces abundant phlegm is probably due mainly to kapha; one that produces yellow or green phlegm with rawness of the throat is most likely due to pitta; and a dry cough, particularly if it is chronic, is usually due to vata.

※ Typical vata symptoms in the body include increased movement (like tachycardia, or the diarrhea of an irritated bowel), decreased movement (like cramps or numbness), perverted movement (like convulsions or tremors), and the separation of one tissue from another (like prolapses, or cracking of the skin).

※ Typical pitta symptoms include indigestion, hot or burning diarrhea, hyperacidity, fever, inflammations, burning sensations, gangrene, ulcerations, bleeding disorders, rashes, jaundice, and anemia.

※ Kapha symptoms include pallor, respiratory congestion, dullness and heaviness of the body and limbs, excessive mucus, itching, and the like.

Sometimes the aggravated doshas cause symptoms on their own, and sometimes they cause them in partnership with ama. Rheumatism and rheumatoid arthritis are conditions in which vata associates itself with ama. When pitta joins forces with ama, its vehicles in the body—such as blood (including menstrual blood) and sweat—become foul-smelling, heavy, thick, and dark. Kapha and ama working together can make mucus sticky, opaque, and ropey, and may cause body aches, insomnia, and other obstructive symptoms.

Ama anywhere in your body will interfere with the free movement of one or the other of vata's subdoshas, but the one whose flow we least like to see disrupted is apana. In fact, apana is more likely than the others to become obstructed, because it has to deal with the large volume of wastes from the food that we continually eat. Whenever any version of vata becomes aggravated it tends either to get stuck (as in constipation or retention of urine), to flow without restraint (diarrhea, urinary incontinence), to create a blockage (like a cyst or fibroid tumor), or to move in the wrong direction. When apana, which is supposed to move downward, heads upward instead, it will pervert progressively whatever previously unperverted subdoshas of vata happen to lie in its path. All sorts of illnesses can result from apana's abnormal upward march, ranging from constipation, bloating, colic and abdominal distention, to heart palpitations, asthma, sinus congestion, and other breathing difficulties. Anywhere that it happens to knot up (back, belly, shoulder, neck, head), apana can create aches.

When apana moves upward it can also create endometriosis, which can produce severe pain during menses. This condition occurs when fragments of endometrium (the uterine lining) travel upward from the uterus into the abdominal cavity, instead of down and out through the vagina as normally happens each month. This tissue can only move upward when apana makes it do so, which apana will do only when its own flow has been reversed.

The Menstrual Season

A healthy menstrual cycle is of paramount importance in many ways to an adult human female's health and well-being. The menstrual cycle is the special benefit that Nature has provided for women to purify their bodies and minds on a monthly basis. Healthy menstruation regularizes a woman's many flows and rhythms, returning her into proper alignment with Nature time and time again; unhealthy menstruation, however, can be very dangerous.

As it is, women today go through many more menstrual cycles during their lives than did the women of earlier days. In the past, a woman usually went through menarche near the end of her teens, quickly became pregnant, and lactated for two to four years after each pregnancy (during which she would not normally menstruate). She thus had little opportunity to go through many cycles. The modern woman, however, goes through menarche earlier (thanks to better nutrition and artificial light) and commonly delivers only one or two children, whom she is usually only able to nurse for a few months at best. She therefore has many more menstrual cycles, during each of which wide hormone swings dramatically affect the tissues of her ovaries, uterus, and breasts. Each of the swings acts as an opportunity for an imbalance to occur, or for an imbalance that already exists to be exacerbated. Some evidence even exists to suggest that a woman's likelihood of developing cancer of the reproductive system increases in relation to the number of her menstrual cycles.

Preserving your menstrual balance is therefore an excellent investment in your future, and the basis of your menstrual balance is, of course, the balance of your doshas. Remember that kapha predominates during the half of the month between the end of the flow and ovulation, during which time the body provides the womb with the best possible nutrients to prepare it to host a child. If pregnancy does not occur, the unused endometrium gradually deteriorates during the pitta half of the cycle (from ovulation until the flow begins), until it becomes a foreign body that the womb must expel. Vata and apana dominate during the days of flow, during which the body appends to the flow all the ama and other filth which has collected in the blood over the course of the month. This "second chance" to purify their blood is probably one reason why women live longer than men. Any previously unnoticed disharmony that may have developed during the month will come into sharp focus just as apana mobilizes to begin its work, which is why you may first notice symptoms of imbalances only when your period begins, or is about to begin.

We must pay special attention to apana, because it is apana that works hard to perform this purification properly. If for some reason the menstrual flow is obstructed, its ama can quickly perfuse the body. Besides endometriosis, ama can cause other imbalances in the reproductive system, such as vaginitis, ovarian cysts, and uterine fibroids; in the rest of the body, it can cause almost anything. As of 1997, more than 150 symptoms all over the body have been attributed to premenstrual syndrome (PMS), and there is every reason to believe that this number will increase. Like any powerful corrective, menses is a two-edged sword. It will most assuredly mobilize your wastes, but what happens to those wastes after they are mobilized will depend on how aligned you and your flows happen to be.

Living with Reality

The need for "living with reality" is nowhere more essential in life than in the context of a woman's menstrual cycle. Nature is not to be denied in her purification quest, and those who will not work with her willingly will find themselves being dragged along in spite of themselves. The schedules we have set for ourselves and the plans we have made are of little interest to Nature, who insists upon following her own agenda. The fact that so many women in our society call menses "the curse" is sufficient indication of how far away from a naturally healthy life we strayed when we took women out of the menstrual hut and told them to work through the month no matter what.

Aside from the emotional nourishment of the camaraderie inside that hut (since women who live in close proximity start to bleed together, many of them would be there at the same time), segregation from society for the two or three days of heavy flow allowed a woman some much-needed rest from her responsibilities. She had time to reflect on and to discuss what had transpired and what was to come, which helped to prepare her for the coming month. Even more important, the powerfully inexorable downward motion of apana helped to remind her of her bond with Mother Earth, the womb from which all of us have taken birth. By renewing this bond, she reactivated her ability to receive the strength and energy from Earth that she would need in the days to come.

When the menstrual hut was banished from our "civilized" society, PMS and various menstrual disorders quickly arose to take its place. Since Ayurveda does not distinguish between the imbalances that happen before the period begins and those that disrupt it, perhaps we should simply call this group of conditions something like "Monthly dysfunction syndrome." The problem is with the entire cycle, not just the portion of it during which you may be miserable, and the remedy lies in returning the entire cycle to harmony. A regular menstrual cycle during your reproductive years provides more than the obvious benefits of greater comfort and balance; it is also a good investment in your future. Some evidence suggests that failing to ovulate every month promotes loss of bone density. Since reduced bone density promotes osteoporosis, and bone density once lost is not easy to replace, preventing that loss is crucial.

Your system has the same four requirements for fertility that a farmer has for a crop: season (rtu), field (kshetra), seed (bija), and juice (rasa). In the context of your body, the season is your cycle; the field is your reproductive organs, and your womb in particular; the seed is your ovum (and, on occasion, the sperm); and the juice is the cocktail of blood, hormones, mucus, and other secretions that fertilize the field and nourish the seed. Some problems with menses can occur due to unhealthiness of seed or juice. Others may arise from change of season, as might happen if you shift your work, study, or sleep patterns, or take a long trip that disorganizes your biorhythms. Field problems include any imbalances or pathologies in your reproductive organs. Any of these factors can be disturbed by any of the three doshas, and in particular if ama is present.

Monthly Dysfunction Syndrome

The following scenarios relate to your condition; your constitution only makes you prone to a similar kind of condition, it does not guarantee it. For example, just because you have a pitta constitution does not mean that you will never have a vata imbalance. In fact, if you permit pitta to make you maniacal in your work or in your play, you may well create a major vata aggravation for yourself.

Vata

Vata creates irregular cycles, or regular cycles in which the spacing between periods is often longer than a month. The flow of blood tends to be scanty, and the blood itself may be unusually thin or may be dark and contain clots. The abdomen may feel tense and rigid. Pain and cramps are common, as is spotting either before or after the main flow. Constipation may develop just before the flow begins, or may have begun during the premenstrual interval. Premenstrual anxiety, interrupted sleep or insomnia, nervous tension, formication (a sensation that ants are wandering over the skin), mood swings, and feelings of "ungroundedness" are common. Sometimes constipation alternates with loose stools.

Women who exercise excessively or who lose too much weight may aggravate their vata so much that they stop menstruating. Some female athletes who lose their periods for this reason also lose so much calcium from their bones that they develop osteoporosis (a characteristically vata-type disease) while still young.

Pitta

Pitta-influenced cycles are usually regular, but they may come close together and there is usually heavy bleeding which lasts for a long time. The blood is usually an intense, bright red, but may also have a bluish, yellowish, or blackish tinge to it. It may produce a sensation of "heat." Occasionally pitta causes reduced flow, especially in emaciated women who have a yellowish tinge to their skin. Pitta women may have loose stools during or just before their periods, and may suffer from medium-strength cramps. Premenstrually, pitta creates irritability, intense food cravings, a burning feeling of excess heat in the body or the mind, acne flare-ups, or skin rashes, or other inflammations, headache (especially migraine), and a vaginal discharge that can be offensive.

Kapha

Kapha excess commonly produces dull pain or cramps during menses. The periods themselves are often regular, with an average quantity of pale, mucus-like blood. Kapha also creates a proneness to water retention, bloating, and swollen breasts, and promotes vaginal itches, yeast infections, stiffness in the back and limbs, slow digestion, and lethargy.

If your cycle is out of kilter, you are likely to find that you have some symptoms from two or perhaps all three of these doshas. This is to be expected; all three doshas work together to create the cycle, and all three can conspire to confuse it. Vaginal discharges, for example, are often due to an excess of kapha that obstructs apana. Fibrocystic breast disease is often a problem of vata (restriction) enveloping kapha.

Remedies

Ayurveda's time-tested approach to treatment is, "Remove the cause, and the effect will disappear." Ayurveda believes that all effects in the organism come from causes, although not according to any sort of synthetic one-cause-creates-one-effect scheme. Ayurveda recognizes that one causative factor can sometimes produce a multitude of effects. You must excise the single cause to remove them. In other situations, where many causes combine to produce a single effect, removal of only one or two of the causes may ameliorate but not extirpate the condition.

Each woman shows her own pattern of causes for menstrual and premenstrual disturbances; some typical ones which can often be eliminated easily include:

- A diet that is inappropriate in quality or quantity for you, in particular, over-consumption of alcohol, meat, caffeine, salt, sugar, and additive-laden junk foods.

- Weak digestion.

- Emotional causes, especially those that involve grief, fear, anger, or shame.

- Insufficient exercise, especially if you are habituated to sleeping during the day.

- Insufficient rest due to over-indulgence in work, sex, travel, exercise, or similar activities.

- Environmental pollutants can stress a woman's reproductive system, particularly during the high-estrogen phase of the cycle.

Other causes may not be easy to remove. Suppose you work the late-night shift in a loud (vata) factory. Your hours cause you to stay up late at night (vata) and sleep during the day (kapha), but quitting is not an option. What do you do? Or suppose you have an infant who wakes up every two hours to nurse, so that your sleep is interrupted (vata). Do you dispense with the baby? No, of course not. What you do in such cases is to work with the external cause as best you can, and otherwise focus on calming the internally aggravated dosha. Causative factors create disease through the medium of the doshas; correct the dosha and you correct the condition.

It is wise to try to decide which dosha is most aggravated (or has the potential to be most aggravated) in you, and to deal with that one first. Begin by asking yourself whether your doshas are balanced. If they are, then you should follow a program that is appropriate for the dosha that is strongest in you constitutionally.

If, however, your doshas are out of balance, ask yourself which dosha seems to be most easily perturbed or pacified by what you eat and what you do. If you can discern a pattern, you will generally find one of the doshas lurking at the center of it. That is the dosha you should focus on first.

If you still cannot decide, then first follow a vata-pacifying program, since apana is the root cause for most menstrual disturbances (and confusion is one of provoked vata's symptoms). You can deal with pitta or kapha thereafter, if there is still a need to do so.

*   Generally speaking, the most important things to do when vata is aggravated are to oil your body, consume soup as your main food in small amounts several times a day, reduce your overall level of activity, practice yoga, tai chi or something similar to balance your energy, and meditate or pray in order to promote internal calmness.

*   Pitta conditions require that you cool your body and mind, eliminate stimulants, consume a pitta-pacifying diet, and learn how to relax.

❋ Kapha requires stimulation, especially in the form of physical exercise, and restrictions on the quantity of food you eat and the amount of time you sleep.

Purification and Palliation

Ayurveda follows a dual approach to treatment: active purification where feasible, otherwise passive purification. Active purification involves preparing the body with oil massage and measured sweating over a number of days, before employing the five purification methods known collectively as *panchakarma*. These include inducing emesis (vomiting) or purgation, administering a medicated enema, or introducing medicines into the nose. Blood-letting is sometimes performed for pitta problems (women with excellent vitality and high pitta can get similar results by donating blood). Purification, which drains "juice" from the bodily field, must also be followed by oiling, and by a period of adequate rest.

Active purification requires the assistance of a trained Ayurvedic specialist, who will know when and how to perform the practices, for improperly administered purifications can create side effects. For example, when the doshas are vitiated in the body without ama, they can be eliminated quickly by purification, but when ama is present, it must first be digested before purification is attempted. Stimulating vata before the channels have been cleared will enrage vata further, and make the obstruction worse. Purification also has its restrictions. It must not be done during extremes of climate—heat waves, cold snaps, flash floods, wind storms—and is forbidden to the very young, very old, very weak, and pregnant women.

While Ayurveda does not hesitate to use surgery and other intensive treatments when mild interventions fail to produce results, it concentrates first on making simple changes in diet and behavior, for simple alterations are sometimes sufficient to produce big results. We will also concentrate on simple measures here. Although all Ayurvedic treatment is (ideally) carefully tailored to the individual and, being health-based, Ayurveda does not prescribe the same treatment for everyone who has the same symptoms, there are many suggestions that are generally good for anyone who wants to improve the "state" of a particular dosha. Why focus on trying either to diagnose or cure Monthly Dysfunction Syndrome, when realigning your state may make that state simply disappear? As it is, none of the current conventional treatments for Monthly Dysfunction Syndrome work any better than a placebo does, and several studies have shown that placebos can work very well. It is better still to have a placebo that realigns and rebalances the body while removing the illness, which is what Ayurveda proposes.

Treating Monthly Dysfunction Syndrome

Every patient suffering from any disease should always be treated as an individual. This maxim holds particularly true for sufferers from Monthly Dysfunction Syndrome, a condition whose symptoms may vary immensely from one woman to the next. With that caveat in mind, we offer here a few general suggestions for promoting a healthy monthly cycle. You may find that merely by implementing one or more of the following recommendations you experience substantial relief, or you may find that even when you abide by them all your imbalance is only assuaged, and not remedied completely. Nevertheless, act on these proposals sincerely and you are certain to derive some degree of benefit.

Get sufficient rest. Although it may not be easy to do, scrounge even a few minutes of repose for yourself here and there. If you can cancel all your activities for the first few days of heavy flow, so much the better; if not, at least reschedule any impending activity that may be stress-inducing. Reduce your normal level of exercise during those days to a minimum; a brief walk is optimal. Avoid cooking—now is the time to get your spouse and kids into the kitchen!

Interiorize. Flow along with your consciousness, wherever it seems to want to take you. Pay more attention to your body consciousness during the flow, opening yourself to any information it wishes to communicate to you about its needs or difficulties. All day long, whether you are working or resting, eating or excreting, focus on breathing slowly, evenly and deep into your abdomen. When you breathe in, let the in-breath drop all the way down into your pelvis and join apana in its downward flow. Breathe out passively, letting apana continue to relax itself downward. Work with apana, and apana will work with you.

Modify your routine. Reduce the amount of time you spend oiling your body, or suspend it altogether for the first few days. During your days of heavy flow take only a brief warm shower, and try to avoid shampooing your head. If apana is very out of balance, you should reduce or postpone your sexual activity (which agitates apana). Pads are preferable to tampons. If you suffer from constipation, you might try aloe vera or triphala, or use a retention enema of oil. For this you will need a small enema syringe, into which you put three ounces of warm oil (sesame, olive, and sunflower are good for vata, pitta, and kapha respectively). When you have inserted the oil, lie down for half an hour or so, until the oil is ready to come out. This will encourage apana's free downward movement and relax both your body and mind.

Eat vata-style. Small meals of warm, mildly spiced, soupy food should be taken frequently during your period. Avoid everything cold and bubbly, and everything heavy (meat, fried foods, most dairy products). Cravings are bound to come your way. Handle them as best you can, perhaps by keeping a mouthful of the food you crave in your mouth as long as you can to extract the most from its flavor. If you crave salt, try eating seaweed, or applying kelp powder to your food instead. If you are able to deal with your salt cravings, you may also be able to reduce vata sufficiently to allow your sugar cravings to dissipate.

If no food seems to be agreeing with you, try *khichadi*, a preparation of split peas cooked with rice. The healthiest of the khichadis is made from mung beans, which are the best of all pulses. They are light, drying, and purifying, and control kapha and pitta without (usually) aggravating vata. A thin soup of split mung with rice is ideal in disease and convalescence, for when mung is cooked with rice it becomes a purifying and nourishing diet which scrapes ama from the body and can be fed safely to almost anyone in almost any state of health. (You can find split mung beans in Indian grocery shops. If you have trouble locating them, sprout some mung beans, wash off the seed coats, and use the sprouts instead.)

BASIC KHICHADI RECIPE

Preparation time: 30 minutes

Makes about 3 servings

1 cup basmati rice

$\frac{1}{2}$ cup mung beans (shelled, split, yellow color)

6 cups boiling water

$\frac{1}{8}$ to $\frac{1}{4}$ tsp turmeric powder

1 pinch asafetida powder

Combine the rice and mung beans and wash twice. Add the mixture to the boiling water, along with the spices. Cook over a medium heat uncovered, until the water is absorbed. Add an additional 1 cup of water. Reduce the heat to low, cover, and cook for 5 more minutes, until this water is absorbed. Additional spices and ingredients should be added at this point, based on whatever imbalances you wish to address (see the chart in appendix 1). The final result should be a stew with a very moist, soft consistency.

Changing your diet

Changing your diet is likely to change your periods. Most of the women I know who have become vegetarians have found that the amount of blood they pass each month was reduced by half once they made the change. Eating meat may sometimes serve you well, of course, such as when your body is emaciated or your strength depleted. In such cases, say the Ayurvedic texts, "meat juice is to be regarded as nectar itself"—not steaks, chops, or hams, but meat broth, especially of chicken or goat. But the less meat you eat, the less you will need to bleed and the better will be your digestion. Anaerobic bacteria (which release toxic waste products) prefer a high-protein diet, while aerobic bacteria (many of which are beneficial) prefer carbohydrates. Meat also putrefies and produces ama faster than other foods, and tends to increase fat rather than flesh unless you exercise strenuously. A vegetarian diet is also better for your bones, as a high-protein diet causes calcium to be lost in your urine.

Eliminating caffeine, at least for the period during which you are trying to regularize apana, can also have dramatic results, especially in women who have fibrocystic breast disease. Reducing or eliminating alcohol can have a dramatic effect on the amount of each month's bloating and water retention, and this effect can be enhanced by cutting back on salt, sour foods, dairy products, and other kapha-creating foods.

Fruit

Some common foods can be pressed into service as remedies for certain monthly complaints. Bananas can help remedy either diarrhea or constipation. While apple pulp or juice will slow diarrhea, stewed whole apples can relax constipation (raw apples tend to increase vata). Ripe mangoes are both laxative and diuretic; they subdue vata, increase the body's strength and cool the blood (unless you eat too many of them). The juice of the sweet variety of pomegranate is digestive, rejuvenative, controls all three doshas, cools the blood, and helps to relieve diarrhea and malabsorption. Sweet grapes also cool the blood, and relieve pitta symptoms like thirst, burning sensations, and fever. If eating grapes doesn't appeal, try holding raisins in your mouth to allay thirst and nausea. Raisins are also good soaked overnight and chewed the next morning, and are particularly good for pregnant women.

Grains

Besides being an easy-to-digest and hypoallergenic food, rice is particularly good for reducing heavy menstrual flow. Take the rice you are going to cook for the day and wash it, once, with water. Catch the water from that wash and drink it, in two or three parts, during the day. If at all possible, drink some tea made from hibiscus flowers along with it (do not make the tea with the wash water). Begin at the end of one period, and stop briefly while you are bleeding during the next one. You can continue this for months on end, if need be. If your body is retaining fluid, tea made from ordinary corntassels is a safe, mild diuretic (organic corn, please—no pesticides!). Barley gruel promotes free urination, reduces pitta, and is much used as a food for convalescents.

Flowers

Roses balance all three doshas, pitta in particular. Gulkand is a preparation made by layering fresh rose petals with honey and sugar and allowing the mixture to mature for two weeks. A teaspoonful or two is taken before bed in water or milk as a mild anti-pitta laxative, especially for the heat of summer; it also helps remedy excessive menstrual bleeding. Rose water is instilled into the eyes to cool them and to control inflammations like conjunctivitis. Rose oil, especially in the form known as attar, is cooling and tonic to the sex organs and the mind. Hibiscus flowers reduce pitta and kapha without aggravating vata. Eaten fresh or made into tea, they remove heat from the body and control bleeding, especially excessive menstrual bleeding. They mitigate the heat of summer and cool the genitourinary tract, purify the blood, and cool the mind. The vegetable okra, which is also a hibiscus species, soothes an irritated digestive tract when eaten boiled.

Spices

Common spices can also help. Cooling, pitta-reducing spices are coriander leaves and fruits and fennel seeds. Some people chew fennel seed after each meal to prevent gas and gallbladder congestion, and its tea alone is sometimes enough to relieve PMS and regularize menstruation.

Sweetened ginger tea can sometimes encourage disturbed or absent menses to regulate themselves. Fenugreek seed improves the digestive, respiratory, and nervous systems, regulates the menses, purifies the skin, and tones the whole organism. Valerian, which balances the three doshas but may aggravate pitta if it is given in excess, is a good sedative, nervine and antispasmodic for menstrual cramps, colic, and digestive upsets. It also digests ama efficiently.

Turmeric is sometimes called "the poor woman's saffron," for it does many of the same things that its more expensive cousin can do. Saffron, which is the collected female reproductive organs of a variety of crocus, is perhaps the supreme spice for the human female's reproductive tract. It regulates the menstrual cycle, relieves dysmenorrhea and PMS, and it promotes fertility, for which purposes it should mainly be used when the woman who is taking it is not bleeding. It is also digestive, and relieves respiratory congestion. Saffron is used in pastes to adorn the skin, to improve the complexion, and to purify the mind. Some texts hail saffron paste as the supreme cosmetic for a woman's breasts.

Chronic Imbalances

"Chronic" comes from a Greek word that means time; common English synonyms for chronic are "habitual" and "usual." The *Journal of the American Medical Association* recently reported that nearly half the people in the United States suffer from at least one chronic illness, and that together these illnesses account for three-quarters of all medical expenditures. Non-steroidal anti-inflammatory drugs (NSAIDs) like ibuprofen, which are the medications of choice for people in chronic pain, cause so many bleeding ulcers (25 percent of those who use NSAIDs in this way develop ulcers) that they are implicated in 10,000 to 20,000 deaths and 100,000 to 200,000 hospitalizations each year. Thus while antacids may relieve the abdominal discomfort that these medicines cause, antacid use doubles the risk of developing a bleeding ulcer.

Although for decades its main emphasis on managing chronic disease was pain relief, the American Medical Association is now actually advising its members to encourage their patients to learn to tolerate pain in certain situations. Lower back pain, for example, is often due to a strain that is something like a sprained ankle and, like a sprained ankle, that back requires rest. When you take painkillers for your sprained back you may feel so much better that you will overdo your physical activity and reinjure your back. This can create yet greater pain for you, and increases the likelihood that the condition will become chronic. Some doctors now also try to reduce the inflammation of rheumatoid arthritis without trying to remove or mask the pain, knowing that as the inflammation dies away, so will the pain.

How Chronic Conditions Develop

Ayurveda welcomes and accepts pain, even while trying to relieve it, for Nature intends pain to be a multi-layered message to us. Underlying the immediate directive—stop using that injured part!—lies a request to look into our lives and see what we are doing to create this misery. When you suppress the pain, you continue to do damage to yourself for as long as the pain's causes continue to operate. Your condition becomes chronic when it remains constant for so long a time that your body-mind-spirit comes to view it as the usual state of things. It has then become a habit of your organism, but it is a malignant habit which creates false flows and can be exceptionally resistant to change. Moreover, if this habit is laid down early enough in life, your body-mind-spirit may retain its memory long after the initial insult has passed.

For example, even though most cases of childhood asthma don't persist into adult life, if you had asthma as a child you are more likely to have it as an adult. That weakness of your respiratory tissue remains in your body memory, waiting for a new cause to trip it off yet again. Another important predictive factor for asthma in adults is having a parent who has a history of asthma—body memory that is transferred from generation to generation. Having previously had more than ten attacks of asthma is also predictive, because the more frequently something happens to the organism, the more likely it is to remember it. A history of eczema is also significant, since the memory of one chronic condition can "re-mind" the organism to develop an entirely different one.

Being female is yet another factor, for more women than men develop asthma as adults. But even if all the predictive factors are positive in your case it is still not definite that you will become asthmatic in your prime. It is only when you allow your life-flow to stray too far from the stream bed that Nature has laid for you that chronic conditions arise. Everything you do to live according to Nature's rules will make asthma's likelihood recede a little further from you, and everything you do that makes your condition deteriorate will draw you a little closer to the edge of the cliff. Once you are on that edge, all sorts of seemingly unrelated stimuli may be able to push you over it. Thunderstorms can trigger asthma attacks, even in people who have never had one. Is it the pollen they stir up, or the mold, or the ions? Is it the tremendous disturbance in the atmospheric vata that they create? Perhaps it is fear of the storm, or the sudden temperature change, or something else altogether. Whatever may be the mechanism, the result is the same: the storm is the impetus, the stimulating factor that throws your own vata into a tailspin.

You cannot rely on being able to fend off all the thunderstorms, literal and figurative, that will arrive through your life. Nor will you always be able to tell what is cause and what effect. In a disease such as rheumatoid arthritis, which comes first—the emotional anguish or the joint inflammation? Other factors are involved, certainly. It also shows a hereditary tendency; it is significantly more severe in cold, damp climates; and women are affected three to five times as often as men. But the emotional component may be most critical. In one path-breaking study of women with a genetic predisposition for rheumatoid arthritis, the majority of those who developed the disease were depressed, alienated, or otherwise emotionally unhealthy.

When you are upset and oppressed by grief, insecurity, fear, or some other powerful emotion, you cannot pay proper attention to what or when you eat, how or when you sleep, with whom or in what way you relate. Your mental anguish seeps right into your tissues, and makes them as rigid and inflexible as your mind. Perhaps one reason why women are more prone to rheumatoid arthritis than men is the degree to which many women resent the dependent role that society foists on them, and the extent to which they feel helpless to do anything about it.

Cancer

Helplessness and hopelessness seem to be important influences in that great medical terror of our time, cancer. Some researchers have proposed a "cancer personality," which is one that refuses to express any negative feelings. The "nice" person who is never obnoxious to anyone, who apologizes for everything, even for being sick, is much more likely to get cancer than someone who lets her feelings show. (Continually feeling angry, of course, is not healthy; it is also a chronic imbalance, and one which predisposes a person to heart disease.) Women who remain calm when the doctor tells them they have a lump that needs to be excised are more likely to have cancer than women who allow themselves to feel what they feel about their potential for harboring a life-threatening disease.

Other causative factors are usually involved, of course. Women have a higher risk of breast cancer if they start menstruating earlier than normal, if they have not had a child by the age of thirty, have had a relative with breast cancer, or eat excess animal fat. Overeating can also be a problem, particularly when much of the food that is ingested is converted into ama. Environmental pollutants are also implicated: "among women having biopsies for removal and diagnosis of suspicious breast lumps, women whose lumps turned out to be cancerous had an average 50 percent higher level of carcinogenic chemicals in their breast fat than those whose lumps were benign." (Lonsdorf et al.)

Fluctuating magnetic and electrical fields can also damage tissues, as can artificial light (rats exposed to light overdose have more breast tumors, and blind women less breast cancer, than the average). Even foundation garments have come in for criticism. One study suggested that women who wear their bras almost twenty-four hours a day are vastly more likely to develop breast cancer than those who wear them for a maximum of twelve hours a day. These women had a greater incidence of breast cancer than did women who wore them for six hours or less per day.

Mentally resilient women to whom a diagnosis of cancer is a challenge are much more likely outlive those who stoically accept their "fate" and go off to die quietly. But fighting the disease is not enough. It is also necessary to learn to be healthy, to submit to Nature, that she may flood you with her healing powers. Laughter is so therapeutic, and thus promotes longevity, because it allows you to take everything, including yourself, a little less seriously. Living with reality is never more essential, and rarely more difficult, than when you have a chronic disease, but reality is usually more palatable when you can laugh about it.

Taking your disease too seriously can be more dangerous than taking yourself too seriously. Ayurveda treats all diseases as actual entities, aliens that invade, possess, and in some cases, come to control their hosts. As your morale drops so does your immunity, and there are diseases waiting around most corners for that chance to possess. Some sufferers make their disease their reality, their security, and their sanity. Deep inside, they so fear that they might disintegrate if they had to relax, feel, weep, and return to face reality that they clutch desperately to their ailments, and refuse to let Nature inside. Nature finds such patients difficult to treat.

Sometimes, though, a forward-thinking woman with a positive outlook has simply been too poisoned by too many toxins for too long for her body to be able to cooperate fully with healing. Such bodies may require the cathartic purification that surgery, chemotherapy, or radiation provides. These are also realities, and if they become your reality, be wise. Strengthen your body before and after your treatments, and make sure you have a good oncologist with a positive outlook. Try to get one who is up on the latest data—one who knows, for example, that women survive breast surgery for cancer nearly twice as well if it is performed during the latter, lower-estrogen half of their menstrual cycle (after ovulation and before flow) than during the earlier, higher-estrogen half. Find one who respects Reality and knows the value of prayer (if you are not aware of the scientifically proven value of prayer, you might want to take a look at *Healing Words* by Larry Dossey, M.D.—see bibliography).

Rejuvenation

After you have gone through a chronic illness, or if your system has been buffeted by the winds of a wild life, rejuvenation is in order. After your body has been purified, select (or have someone select for you) a rejuvenating substance that agrees with both your constitution and condition, and consume it each morning for a minimum of 40 days before you try to evaluate its efficacy in your system. Many of the herbs described in this book are rejuvenative, including aloe vera, shatavari, ashvagandha, licorice, bala, shilajit and chandra prabha. Chyvanaprasha continues to be beneficial in adulthood, especially when it is prepared with substantial amounts of saffron, which renews and revitalizes the female reproductive system.

Taken internally, triphala rejuvenates the "internal skin" of your digestive tract, and if applied externally would rejuvenate your outer skin as well. Ayurveda's *Sharngadhara Samhita* notes that with each passing decade the body loses, one by one, childhood, growth, luster, complexion, intelligence, and skin health. This means that if you are not attentive to your organism, your complexion and your skin's luster will have dulled significantly by the end of your twenties, the intelligence of your body-mind-spirit will have dimmed by the end of your thirties, and by the age of fifty your skin will have lost its vitality. A healthy body breathes through its skin as well as through its lungs, therefore, keeping your skin healthy can help to keep the rest of you in good shape. To this end, daily oil application to the body is a must, combined with regular massage by an expert. Oil is food for your skin, and creams containing rejuvenative herbs that agree with your dosha may be considered its drink. Keep your skin regularly moisturized and well oiled and it will remain supple, intelligent, and healthy long past its potential expiration date.

Rejuvenation is not by substance alone, though. Substances work best when combined with behavior modification, particularly with respect to life's three pillars: sleep, food and sex.

Sleep

Sleeping during the day for longer than a nap is permissible only when you are very weak or exhausted, or in very hot weather; otherwise, day sleep increases kapha and clogs the channels. Staying up all night long increases vata and decreases kapha. It is wise to try to go to sleep during the four hours or so immediately post-sunset, which kapha (which promotes sleep) rules. If you stay up after 11 P.M. pitta will kick in, which will make it difficult for you to sleep easily or deeply thereafter. Also, if you go to sleep early you will be ready to wake up during the predawn hours, during which the naturally increased vata will promote excretion of everything that must be excreted. If you have a habit of sleeping late, try working your way backward half an hour per week over several weeks, until your bedtime is back within the kapha envelope.

Food

Everyone eats, but not everyone eats healthily. If we are truly to begin to rejuvenate ourselves through food, we need to examine not merely what we eat but also how we eat it. The aim is not to become fixated on your diet, or to be obsessed about what you could or should be doing differently—instead, your goal is to create healthy eating patterns in both mind and body. These habits can then serve by their example to teach other parts of you how to create and maintain the health that comes about by being able to digest and utilize every stimulus that comes your way.

Rules for Healthy Eating

1. **Eat foods whose qualities agree with you.** The first place to look for agreement is in the food's taste. Because children are growing they love the sweet taste—sweet promises nutrition to the body, which means that children should be eating sweet foods that are nutritious for them. But sweet is also the heaviest of the tastes, and must be balanced by judicious quantities of the other five according to constitution, season, and other relevant factors. Our concern is that sweetness be produced within the body, which may mean that the child will sometimes have to eat things that are not sweet in order to create sweetness.

   Beef, pork, and milk are examples of foods that are innately heavy for digestion; mung beans, venison, and rice are innately light. You can safely eat your fill of food that is light, but heavy food should never form more than half your meal. Do not eat heavy or kapha-producing food (like melons, yogurt, sesame products, cheese or ice cream) after sunset. In general, raw food is heavier than cooked, and preserved food is heavier than fresh.

Deep-fried food, which aggravates all three doshas and impairs the eyesight, should not be eaten regularly. Avoid all ice-cold food and drinks, and products that contain cooked honey.

How much you should eat depends on your stomach capacity, which refers in Ayurveda not to the size of your stomach but to the strength of your digestive fire. You can safely eat that amount of food which you will punctually digest without any disturbance. At any one meal, it is ordinarily best to fill your stomach one-third full of solid food and one-third full of liquid food, leaving the last third empty to permit free stirring. Pitta people, who usually have an intense digestive fire, often have cast-iron stomachs (at least early on in their lives). The kapha digestive fire is less intense but equally regular, which means that kapha people can generally get by with more dietary misdeeds than can the vata type, whose digestive fire is so irregular that it often dies away for no apparent reason.

It is wise to eat food whose qualities oppose the qualities of the climate and season in which you live. This means that consuming, say, yogurt and cheese during a Glasgow or Seattle winter would be as unwise as eating a big plate of fried fish smothered in garlic during a San Antonio or Panama City summer. Some foods produce different effects in the body with changes of season or climate; yogurt, for instance, increases pitta when taken in the hot season, but aggravates kapha during the cold season.

A food's qualities can be altered by the way in which it is prepared. Rice, which is naturally light, can be made even lighter by puffing it, and puffed rice can be made heavy by mixing it with marshmallow cream. Milk becomes lighter when it is heated with spices like saffron, and rice becomes heavier when it is cooked with milk. Refrigerated food becomes heavier, as does food preserved by other methods.

Most people, at least initially, should focus their diets around whole grains, as have many traditional cultures. Thus a typical peasant meal on most continents consists of a larger quantity of grain served with a smaller quantity of pulses or of meat, vegetables, and other supplementary substances.

Combining different foods generally makes the resulting mixture heavier, unless they have been cooked together. Food combining is more important for vata people than for other types because the vata digestive tract is unable to handle too great a variety of food at one time, no matter how small the quantity. Vata people therefore do best on one-pot meals: soups, stews, and the like, in which all the ingredients lose their own individuality and are melded into a single substance. One-pot meals are best for everyone during illness, convalescence, and rejuvenation therapy.

2. **Eat "living" food.** Overcooked, undercooked, burnt, bad-tasting, unripe, overripe, putrified, stale, or just revolting food is dead food. Refrigerated food is near death, especially if it has already been cooked once. It is better to avoid leftovers, for freshness of mind and spirit requires the sort of freshness of body that comes from eating fresh food. If you must eat leftovers, heat them up, and avoid mixing fresh food with them.

   Raw food is more "alive" than cooked food, in the sense that its prana is more intact. But it is also more difficult to digest than cooked food, and only those whose digestive fires are exceptionally strong should eat large amounts of raw food. Most people do best on a steady diet of warm, well-cooked, unctuous, fresh food. Eating habits also affect digestive capability; thus if you are used to cooked food, you will find raw food particularly difficult to digest because your system is not used to it.

3. **Antidote a food's negative qualities.** The basis of traditional Indian cuisine is the antidoting of possible food side effects with appropriate preparation. For example, fish is often cooked with fennel or coconut milk, or is served with lemon to cool it and make it less likely to aggravate pitta. Turmeric is always added when beans or lentils are cooked, for a similar reason. Pulses are

also cooked with oil, with something sour like tamarind, and with spices such as ginger, garlic, and asafetida to prevent vata disturbance.

More Guidelines for Healthy Eating

- Eat only after the previous meal has been digested. Healthy kapha types should eat at most twice a day, allowing at least a six-hour gap between meals. They should not snack. Pitta people can eat three meals daily with gaps of four to six hours between them, and may snack if they retain a consistent four-hour gap. Most vatas should eat small meals three or four times a day, and may snack as needed with gaps of at least two hours.

- Eat nothing at night within two hours of going to bed.

- Don't cook for yourself alone. The gift of food is the best gift of all. Before you begin to eat, try to feed someone else—a pet, a plant, a neighbor. This is a practical way of thanking Nature for her food. In India, it was once common to make a five-fold offering of food before eating: to the home cooking fire, a cow, a crow, a dog and a stranger. This may not be feasible at every meal, but the more often you do it, the more your children will be able to enjoy the particular sweetness that comes from feeding someone.

- Sit to eat, whenever possible facing east, in a congenial, clean, well-decorated, quiet place, either alone or with people whom you find agreeable, after washing your hands and face.

- Immediately before you begin to eat, chew some ginger marinated in lemon or lime juice to awaken your taste buds, to start your juices flowing, and to purify your tongue and mouth. (Pitta types and people with pitta provocations should omit this step.)

※ Feed all five senses. Look at the food and appreciate its appearance and aroma before you begin; listen to the sounds it makes, especially while it is cooking. Chew each morsel slowly and attentively many times, to extract its flavor thoroughly. When feasible, eat with your hands, so that your skin and your brain can enjoy the food's temperature and texture.

※ Generally, it is best to drink nothing but warm water with your meal, and that in small sips.

※ Eat neither hurriedly nor slowly, but concentrate on and appreciate the qualities of the food you are eating. Eat without laughing or talking much (you may find sooth-ing music agreeable), and without television, radio, or other intrusive media to distract your attention.

※ Do not eat when you are not hungry, and do not fail to eat when you are hungry.

※ Do not eat when you are angry, depressed, bored, or otherwise emotionally unstable, or immediately after physical exertion. Keep as large a gap as possible be-tween meals, and certainly not less than two hours.

※ Stroll about a hundred steps after a meal, to assist the digestive process, but do not exercise, enjoy sex, study, or sleep within an hour of eating. You may, however, relax, lying on your left side to aid the functioning of the right nostril, which will encourage good digestion.

※ Never waste food.

Prayer

The most important of all the rules of eating is to pray over your meal. Give thanks to the Creator for the food you offer into your digestive fire. Food is the prana, the life force, of living beings; our lives are a continual search for food. In the words of a Sanskrit proverb, "life lives off life"—we maintain our own lives by consuming other living beings. All living beings possess their own awareness and feelings, whether or not they can communicate them to us. The act of sincerely thanking the Creator for the sacrifice our food has made for us, allows the Creator to align the flow of the food's awareness properly with our own. This is particularly true when you are praying over food in a restaurant, or food that has been cooked by someone who does not have your best interests at heart. Sadly, the most negative qualities a food can possess are the negative emotional qualities that a misguided chef can contribute to what he or she prepares. Whenever possible, you should ensure that whoever is cooking for you is someone who loves you dearly.

Most of us learn to mumble or race through grace as we sit hungry at our parents' table, but too few of us learn to make those words count. It is easier to do that over the stove than over a plate—which cook has never sent up a petition to the unseen powers to keep the soufflé from falling or to get the bread to rise? It is easy to project love and nourishment into the food you cook, and to provide others with the opportunity to do the same. As a parent, you may not be able to teach your children how to cook, or how to love, but you can create conditions for them in which they will have the chance to learn how essential love and good food are to a healthy, happy life.

Addiction

If only all our peculiar behaviors would disappear as easily as unhealthy sleep patterns. Sadly, most dependencies that we create for ourselves are unlikely to vanish automatically. Our society is full of addictions, because we try to find on the outside what can really only be found within. It is very easy to become addicted to food, because food itself is an addiction, a necessary dependence on substances from outside ourselves to perpetuate our embodied life. Everyone is searching for sweetness, and if you lack sweetness in your daily life it will be very tempting to search for it in your food.

Many people become addicted to foods that give them what they think they need. Vata people love sugar, which temporarily provides instant stimulation and satisfaction. Pitta people tend to go for meat, alcohol, and fatty, salty, sour, and spicy foods, which make them more intensely driven. Kapha people search out heavy or fatty foods, which reinforce their natural complacency. All of us use our food to affect our consciousness, but many of us use food to reinforce our mental proclivities, and let our minds convince us that the things they like are also good for our bodies. It is better to work to improve these proclivities by consciously selecting those tastes and other qualities that will help you balance your doshas. The simple act of gaining control over your diet can also provide you with the discipline to control many more aspects of your behavior, because you are what you eat. Every food you eat contributes to your self-awareness and your awareness of the world around you.

Occasional fasting helps control food addictions, purifies the body, rests the digestive organs, normalizes and heightens the mouth's taste sense, and encourages a more reverential approach to the act of eating. Living on a monodiet (a single food or beverage) for one day twice a month or one day a week is a good way to fast. Those who are more balanced may get better results from living on water alone, or even by doing without water at all, on that day. Ayurveda generally frowns on longer fasts—which are popular in some circles in the West—for physical purification, because they encourage degeneration of the body's tissues and loss of cohesion between body and mind.

As you get used to limiting your eating for one day on a regular basis, your mind is likely to feel less threatened by the idea of giving up one of your addictions. When you do find yourself used to an unhealthy food you should eliminate it gradually, to permit your system to adjust. The Ayurvedic texts speak of eliminating the offending food by reducing its amount gradually over a week, but since people today are more intensely addicted to more foodstuffs than ever before, the modern body usually needs more than a week to adjust. Food can become as much a substance of abuse as any narcotic, and eating can involve cravings as intense as drugtaking. As with drugs, cues activate the cravings; thus a chocoholic's body can learn to react as strongly to the sight of a chocolate wrapper as rats who are sensitized to morphine injections react to a needle that has no drug in it.

Eliminating an addiction is rarely easy, and may require professional guidance. When feasible, though, gradual removal of an addiction is far better for your balance than is yanking it suddenly from your life. For one thing, when you become habituated to a food, your system learns how to cope with its negative effects, knowing that you will be eating it regularly. When you are addicted you still experience such negative effects, but less acutely; they accumulate in the body and wait for an opportunity to express themselves, which they may well try to do as you try to give up that food.

Antidotes

While you wait for your organism to be ready to relinquish its attachment, you can at least antidote that food. The negative effects of most foods can be reduced (although not eliminated) by consuming that food with its antidote. Melons go well with black pepper, for example, because it dries up their heavy wateriness before this can increase kapha; many spices, including cinnamon, can do the same things for yogurt. You can add cardamom to your coffee in the same way that the Arabs do, to reduce the effects of its acidity, and drink carrot juice to help ameliorate the side effects of alcohol.

Eating sweets releases endorphins within you, increasing your pain tolerance. Chronic pain patients sometimes permit themselves to eat a diet of sweets alone, although these will eventually produce side effects such as hypoglycemia and diabetes. Karavellaka (*Momordica charantia,* a very bitter cucumber-like vegetable available in Asian groceries as Chinese bitter melon) is popular among some Indian and Chinese diabetics, who eat it in order to control their blood sugar. Karavellaka can thus act as an antidote to sweets, and as a medicine for sweet overdose; but if you continue to overconsume sweets while you eat karavellaka it may only be able to postpone, not prevent, metabolic breakdown. Do not forget the words of the *Charaka Samhita:* "Even food, which is the life of living creatures, if taken in an improper manner destroys life, while poison, which by nature is destructive of life, if taken in the proper manner acts as an elixir." Most food addictions eventually poison you; it is just a matter of time.

ADDICTION AND TASTE

A food addiction is really a taste addiction, for certain foods indisputably taste better to each of us than do others. While Ayurveda has always maintained that the internal reality of the outwardly ephemeral taste is very real to the tasting organism, there is as yet no practical, "scientfic" way to verify externally this internal perception. However, scientific evidence is now accumulating in support of this principle. One researcher has discovered, for example, that the mere taste of fatty food in the mouth (even if it is not swallowed) causes the concentration of fat in the blood to surge.

Fat and Dieting

Fat is a major concern for a vast majority of us. More than 70 percent of American women say they feel fat, even though only 23 percent of them are actually overweight. Anorexia and bulimia are only the fast-cycling manifestations—in identity they conform to our fast-paced, vata-provoked world—of what dieters have been doing in slower succession for centuries: overeating as a proxy for what they think they are missing from their lives, then undereating when they become alarmed by the changing shapes of their bodies.

Although there is little doubt that being overweight is unhealthy, few women realize that repeated dieting will in the long term make them fatter. For one thing, although people love to blame their bodies for their lack of impulse control, the body's consciousness is much too sensible ever to starve itself. Starvation is what the body most fears, and since it has only a limited capacity to store carbohydrates, none to store proteins, and an almost unlimited capacity to store fat, fat is what it will store when it gets a chance. Moreover, dieting drives down your metabolism, making it harder to burn off calories, and encourages you to eat more once you go off the diet. Dieting can also be dangerous to your long-term health, because dieters who swing through cycles of weight loss and gain run a higher risk of dying from heart disease than do those whose weights remain approximately stable, even if they are overweight.

Today's "anti-diet" movement is certainly an improvement over the well-entrenched "dieting-to-excess" cult. Even so, anti-dieting does not address the real cause of the problem. It just makes women feel better (or lets them convince themselves that they feel better) about being overweight. Let us turn the statistic around. If more than 70 percent of American women say they feel fat, and only 47 percent are deluding themselves, then 23 percent of American women—one-quarter of the entire population of female adults in that society—are overweight.

Ayurveda classifies obesity, gout,m and diabetes among the "diseases of affluence," the affluent state of mind being one in which a person believes she has time and/or money to waste. It is just this sort of perceived affluence that puts on weight. An Ayurvedic text comments: "Boredom, mindless entertainment, continuous eating, and oversleeping: these will fatten you up just like a hog." Most of us have experienced the truth of this saying during the holidays: Liberated from drudgery, we stuff ourselves like pigs, watch television until we become bored and indolent, and drift off into dreamland. This is an infallible way to gain weight; repeated regularly, it leads to obesity.

Self-transformation

Starving the body to punish the mind is not the answer. Nor is indulgence—remember the blood lipid surge that comes from the mere taste of fatty food in the mouth? Taste makes waste. The answer to all "diseases of affluence" is healthy austerity—that is, a healthily austere state of mind. Austerity does not require self-flagellation, or grim renunciation of pleasure. Austerity is the recognition that waste of any kind is wasteful, particularly in the context of your body. Your body has to deal with the nutrients and the wastes from your food; this gives your body, not your mind, priority over what goes into you, and when.

As soon as you transfer control of your diet to your body, by making the commitment to let your body run the nutrition show, your body will begin to cooperate with you to transform itself. Therefore, if you are overweight, then your goal should be to transform yourself, and not just to lose weight. This is a slower process, but in weight loss, as in all other aspects of medicine, haste makes waste. Reducing your weight is a part of self-transformation which needs to occur gradually and consistently if it is to be permanent.

The first step in self-transformation is to balance your doshas, which you can begin to do by a gradual change to a diet that is appropriate for your condition. To go on a strict anti-kapha diet and exercise program when you are highly vata-provoked could throw you even further off balance. Work with your body, and let your mind sit quietly for a change. That way, it might learn something.

Remember also that your ideal weight will be one which is appropriate for your constitution. Women blessed with a kapha constitution should not waste their time (or their bodies) trying for the anorexic, magazine-model look. Even though it is generally better to be too thin than too fat, having insufficient fat for your body type will weaken your immunity. Fat is good for you, in the proper amount; hatred of fat is self-hatred. Forget about fat; think instead about recreating yourself.

Food as Medicine

Even if you move gradually into a lifestyle that promotes health, it is still possible sometimes to find yourself unbalanced. As your body relinquishes its previous alignments, temporary misalignments may arise. Ayurveda believes it is always best to begin with the simplest, mildest treatment for a disease, particularly when that disease has arisen as the body purifies itself. If dietary change is the most fundamental treatment for most diseases, the therapeutic use of spices is only slightly less fundamental. As part of our daily food, spices promote the digestion of the food they are cooked with, and when used remedially they promote the digestion of ama, which is made up of food that you previously ingested.

The following are a few of the ways in which simple spices can make a difference to your health:

- A tea made of equal parts of cumin, coriander, and fennel is a mild, effective way to improve your digestive fire. A teaspoon of roasted cumin powder chewed at bedtime does something similar, but is slightly more warming. Anyone can chew cardamom pods for the same purpose, but only vata or kapha types should regularly chew caraway or anise. Caraway or anise decoction can help to relieve colicky pain or stomach cramps. Anise, dill, fennel, and fenugreek increase the production of breast milk, and medicate the milk to strengthen the baby's digestion. Dill seeds relieve gas, colic, and hiccup, and are even good for small children; with fenugreek, dill controls diarrhea. Cardamom and coriander seed are both tonic to the kidneys and bladder.

❧ Cayenne powder makes good first aid for animal bites (it will sting!), and for acute diarrhea that really must be stopped quickly (as in cholera). A teaspoonful taken with hot water (or, better still, hibiscus tea) will quickly stop acute intestinal or uterine bleeding long enough for you to get to a doctor. However, repeated use for these purposes (and for diarrhea) will aggravate the problem the cayenne is given to solve by provoking pitta further. Ginger, garlic, and onions also tend to be pitta-provoking.

❧ Garlic relieves vata and kapha, improves digestion, appetite, circulation, and tissue nutrition, kills harmful bacteria without destroying useful ones, promotes memory, and is useful in dry skin diseases, parasites, colic, cough, heart disease, asthma, and indigestion. Garlic has been used to cure or improve cases of typhoid, diphtheria, whooping cough, pneumonia, bronchitis, bronchiectasis, influenza, and tuberculosis, to reduce cholesterol and to scavenge heavy metals from the tissues. It decreases high blood pressure and body and joint pain, and is said to assist parents in conceiving an intelligent child.

❧ Onions stimulate the heart, promote bile production, and reduce blood sugar. The fresh juice of one medium-sized red onion makes a good heart tonic when consumed in the morning with 1 tablespoon of raw honey. Smelling a crushed onion can sometimes cure headache or relieve nausea. In various combinations, onions have been employed for allaying conditions such as asthma, laryngitis, diarrhea, dysentery, kidney stones, retention of urine, hemorrhoids, amenorrhea, mammary abscess, heat stroke, and rheumatism.

❧ While dried ginger controls and balances all three doshas (although in excess it may increase pitta), fresh ginger can increase pitta and is forbidden in conditions when pitta is high (such as heavy bleeding, inflamed skin diseases, and fevers). Ginger inflames the appetite, intensifies the digestive fire, relieves bloating and abdominal distention due to gas, prevents motion sickness, and (with rock salt and cumin in water after meals) relieves chronic diarrhea. With lime juice and sugar or salt it is a popular Indian first-aid remedy for sunstroke. Ginger is Ayurveda's supreme toxin-digester; a weak tea of powdered ginger is a good way to help digest ama that has accumulated in your gut, and its strong tea with castor oil is used for rheumatism and rheumatoid arthritis. Ginger promotes circulation, especially when applied to the body. Ginger baths promote warmth, and help relieve musculoskeletal aches and pains (start with a tiny amount, say 1 tablespoon, in a silk or rayon bag, with an equal amount of bicarbonate of soda; increase the quantity slowly). A paste of powdered ginger on the forehead relieves some kinds of headache (don't leave it on too long). Consumed with turmeric in hot milk, dry ginger loosens and liquifies thick respiratory congestion; for productive cough, it is used alone or with black pepper and long pepper (*Piper longum,* available in many Indian grocery stores), with honey. For dry cough, pharyngitis, bronchitis, nausea, and vomiting, fresh ginger juice is used with mint juice, lemon juice, and honey. In influenza, fresh ginger juice is often given with fenugreek decoction and honey. Dry ginger and jaggery (solidified sugarcane juice; you can also use molasses) make urine and feces flow more freely.

One spice which is not yet too common in the West is asafetida, which you can find in diluted form in Indian grocery shops under the name "hing." Asafetida is exceptionally pungent, hot, and foul-smelling, and cures vata and kapha while increasing pitta. Its strongest action is to free the downward movement of apana; the *Charaka Samhita* says that no other herb is better for this purpose. One way to take it is to mix hing in equal parts with the powders of turmeric, ginger, caraway seed, cumin, and coriander. You can take $1/8$ teaspoon of this mixture, combined with enough honey to make a paste, and wash it down with a little cumin-coriander-fennel tea as often as every half-hour, to help apana release itself. You may also be able to locate hingvashtaka churna, which is a compound of asafetida that is similar to the above asafetida mixture and is used the same way, for indigestion, colic, and other ailments caused by an inhibited apana.

Fenugreek tea promotes sweating (especially in fevers like influenza, which are due to vata and kapha), purifies breast milk, is decongestant, and improves dysentery and arthritis. Unless you are very pitta-provoked, you can take $1/4$ teaspoon of a mixture of 4 parts cardamom, 3 parts fenugreek, 2 parts ginger, and 1 part each cinnamon, black pepper, and bay leaf. Add enough honey to make a paste, and lick the paste slowly when you have a cough, cold, or other upper-respiratory congestion. Fenugreek is given with valerian for insomnia and neuroses. The seeds are made into a confection in India and given to women after childbirth to strengthen them and to promote milk production, and the seed paste is applied externally to boils and abscesses.

Nutmeg and mace are used more or less interchangeably to calm the nerves of the lower abdomen. They control acute diarrhea, and assist with control of dysentery and other intestinal dysfunctions. They can be given with buttermilk for diarrhea or with milk to induce sleep and control premature ejaculation. Nutmeg powder has also been used in urinary incontinence, and it is an ingredient in many aphrodisiac mixtures.

🕉 Turmeric, which balances the three doshas, is used externally and internally to purify both blood and mind. Every dish of dal (simmered and pureed legumes) cooked in India has turmeric added to it, to keep the blood cool. Applied to wounds, it slows bleeding; its paste is used on bruises, bites, stings, open wounds, boils, and breast disorders, and with sandalwood to purify and beautify the skin (brides and grooms in India are anointed with this mixture before they are wed). It is used in eyedrops for conjunctivitis, and its smoke is employed in fainting, hiccups, and asthma. As a natural antibiotic, it protects rather than destroys the intestinal flora, and it promotes the production of bile. It is effective, in combination, in the control of diabetes and in several types of skin disease.

Sex and Relationships

Virilization *(vajikarana)* is one of the two limbs of the tree of Ayurveda that have no direct analogue with the branches of modern medicine (the other being *rasayana,* rejuvenation). Virilization is both rejuvenation for your reproductive organs and "prejuvenation" for your children. It is a way to select healthy genes with which to create a child with a healthy constitution, initiating a health progression that will bear delicious fruit in both your children and their descendants.

No contraception is perfect, which means that every act of sexual intercourse between two fertile partners has the potential to produce a child. When you elect to enjoy coitus with a fertile man you should therefore be sure that the man with whom you sleep is one whose child you are willing to bear. You should also be in the right mood, and in the right place if you are trying to conceive a child; conceptional sex is too valuable an experience to relegate to the back seat of a car, a pool table, or the undergrowth in the local park (the rules for recreational sex are a little looser...).

The purpose of virilization is to strengthen the bodies of the couple involved, that they may create in themselves maximal excitement at the moment of congress. This is because some of the joy and excitement that flows through a blissful sexual experience can be transmitted directly into the sperm and ovum, and when these two cells unite to form a zygote—which is the first cell of a fetus—that joy provides a foundation of satisfaction which can persist lifelong.

The physical basis of blissful sex is physical health; your reproductive juices gain optimal qualities only when all your other tissues are happy and well fed. Virilization sometimes implies the use of aphrodisiacs, only a few of which are for arousal. Most are meant to nourish directly the reproductive juices. One example of an aphrodisiac drink is hot milk into which nutmeg, ginger, ashwagandha, shatavari, bala, licorice, and saffron have been mixed and into which a small amount of shilajit has been dissolved. Chandra prabha is one example of an aphrodisiac pill, and garlic, onions, and ginger are good examples of aphrodisiac foods. Onion juice, for example, when taken mixed with honey, ginger juice and ghee, is said to increase the sexual juices immediately.

Aphrodisiacs do not work well on their own; they require a healthy field in which to do their work. While part of what makes for a healthy field is nutrition (putting things into the body), another part is preservation—making sure that you do not lose too much juice from your body. Diarrhea and hemorrhage are two ways of losing juice; excessive sex is another. Although it is no longer a popularly accepted concept, too-frequent orgasm does not promote healthy body-mind-spirit integration. Fortunately for women, orgasm's sudden discharge of tremendous energy is more disturbing to a man's nervous system than it is to a woman's. To protect their ojas, Ayurveda advises men to ejaculate a maximum of three times a week in the mildest season of the year, and not more than twice a month in climatic extremity. Ejaculation should be avoided entirely immediately after meals and during acute disease or convalescence. Although no limit is put on a woman's orgasms, both sexes are advised to follow a post-orgasmic regimen to prevent vata disturbance. This includes urination (to regulate the activity of apana), cleaning of the face, teeth, and body (to free the passage of vata and prana on its surface), and mild stretching (for the same purpose).

Male and Female Orgasm

Loss of ojas, which is the root cause of much sexual stress, is often caused by sexual overindulgence, which itself is often caused by mutual sexual misunderstanding. The male and female orgasms are physiologically similar, to the extent that some women even ejaculate a clear and copius fluid (called in Ayurveda "female semen"), but psychologically, psychically, and in every other way, the orgasms of the two sexes are quite different. The reflex path of a man's orgasm ends in his limbic system, which is part of the ancient R-brain. "R" is for reptile, and male sexual response has not changed all that much since the days when reptile males were the planet's hot studs. The male orgasm is a linear physical response. When a man becomes aroused he is as ready to leap into bed and go to work as he is ready to leave again once he has completed his task. No emotional connection to his physical response is necessary at all.

For most women, the situation is precisely the opposite. They must have some sort of emotional response in order for their physical response to flow freely. A woman's every orgasm differs somehow in quality from the ones before and after it (or at least they should); a man has the same orgasm time and time again, differing only in the intensity of his arousal before his discharge.

This is one salient reason why the average man is totally in the dark when it comes to comprehending female sexual response. Men think in terms of linear cause and effect. "If this woman is lubricating, she must be aroused; if she doesn't feel aroused, her feelings must be wrong, because physiology does not lie." Another reason lies with the clitoris, which Masters and Johnson called "a unique organ in the total of human anatomy" because its sole purpose is to provide pleasure. They also noted wryly that "the human female frequently is not content with one orgasmic experience," and suggested that when it comes to the clitoris, women get "frustrated by male ineptitude" (quoted by Sallie Tisdale). It is no wonder that some women find sex with other women superior to sex with men, or that other women have enumerated the many ways in which a cucumber is preferable to a man. For the average person, all sex is masturbation. The partner's body is merely the object through which he or she enjoys a pleasure that is wholly internal.

Sexual Satisfaction

Couples who fail to take the time to understand sex, and one another, achieve at best some self-gratification rather than mutual satisfaction. Attempting to compensate for dissatisfaction with frequent, obsessive sex only makes the problem worse. For one thing, extremely vigorous sex can raise the blood pressure to a point where it causes tiny blood vessels to burst and tissues to tear in the eyes; this can cause blurred vision for months. Nor is sleeping around the answer. Research from Johns Hopkins reports that thanks to human papilloma virus, women whose husbands have had more than 21 sex partners in their lives are 11 times more likely to get cervical cancer than other women; the wives of men who frequent prostitutes have a likelihood that is eight times greater.

Unsatisfying sex is a major destroyer of ojas, and loss of ojas weakens your aura. Indiscriminate sexual activity with a multitude of partners fragments your aura further. The more fragmented your aura, the less you will be willing (or psychically able) to let someone inside you in anything more than a physical sort of way. For a man, and for some women, this situation may be quite tolerable. In this way, prostitutes and men are made for one another— they exchange money for the purchase of a physical act of sex, not a psychological one. But most women do not find this sort of sexual activity at all satisfying, and unsatisfactory sex thus becomes the cause of much disease among today's women. First it disturbs the monthly cycle, then it disrupts the rest of the organism.

Moreover, should such an unsatisfied woman become pregnant, her misery will be transferred to the child in her womb by the toxins circulating in her impure blood. Any baby grown in such an environment will grow up dissatisfied and angry, with those emotions at the foundation of her constitution. A zygote that was infused with some of the immense satisfaction that a couple feel at the moment of a satisfying orgasm will develop into a child who will be more easily satisfied with life than will a child whose parents were convulsed by powerfully twisted emotions at the time of conception. Such parents leave their child instead with a constitutional hunger that she will always find difficult to satiate.

The parents themselves will also be left unfulfilled, because they are searching in all the wrong places for sweetness. If, instead of persisting in continuing along a path that is leading them nowhere, they were to take the time and effort needed to develop healthy sexual lives, they would be able to extract a profound degree of lasting sweetness from their sexual relationship.

Les Différences

A useful first step toward sexual satisfaction is to realize, once and for all, that women differ from men. "Vive la différence!" we might add, echoing that Frenchman who roared his opinion during a debate some years ago on the floor of France's National Assembly. One difference is staying power. While 125 male fetuses are conceived for every 100 female ones, at birth the male-to-female ratio has decreased to 105:100. By age seventy-five, 65 males compete for the attentions of every 100 females; at age eighty-five, only 40 men remain for each 100 women.

Women perceive the world differently. Their hearing is more sensitive than men's (they seem to use both ears, while men seem to rely on the right ear), and in conversation they are more attentive to emotional messages—overt and subliminal—than are men. Part of the distinction is structural: the corpus callosum, a structure which connects together the right and left hemispheres of brain, is 25–40 percent larger in a woman than in a man, which suggests that women are naturally better able than men to integrate their many brain functions. Also, the brains of the sexes seem to be formatted differently for pain, for certain opiates (kappa opoids) have a very positive analgesic effect on women, but very little effect on men.

Hormones

Women are more sensitive than men to touch, taste, and smell. Perhaps this is why pheromones, the hormone odors contained in the sweat of both sexes, also seem to affect women more than men. Male pheromones help to regularize a woman's menstrual cycle, and women who live together usually develop synchronized menstrual periods through the effect of their own pheromones on each other. The sex hormones also create some differences. The male hormone testosterone seems to affect the development of right-brain function, tending to make the brain more specialized and less integrated. Thus men excel at spatial reasoning (a right-brain function) and women at abstract reasoning, although women improve their spatial rotation scores by 50–100 percent during menstruation (when their estrogen levels are lowest), and men improve their scores in spring (when their testosterone is highest).

Women whose testosterone levels are usually high (some women produce ten times as much testosterone as others) are usually more sexually active—and claim to enjoy sex more—than those whose levels are normal. Their sexual desire and activity fluctuate wildly, however, with their highest levels of testosterone occuring at mid-cycle. Mid-cycle is when an ordinary woman's desire peaks; high-testosterone women tend to become most aroused just before and just after their menstrual periods. Alcohol boosts the amount of testosterone in a woman's bloodstream, especially at ovulation (and if she is on the Pill), thus making her more amorous; by contrast, in men, excess alcohol depresses testosterone. Alcohol makes a poor aphrodisiac choice for women, though, because they absorb more alcohol and become intoxicated more quickly than do men who have drunk the same amount (they also metabolize nicotine more slowly than men).

High-testosterone women tend to like fast-paced, demanding careers, they complain more about sexual frustration, and are less likely to be married to, or living with, a man than are normal-testosterone women. Testosterone has also been correlated with aggressive behavior, especially in young males, while female hormones tend to produce opposite results; male rats given estrogen and progesterone became model mothers. Although hormones cannot explain every male-female difference, they may well lie at the root of the pithy formulae which surface now and again to express these differences. "Men are creatures of ambition," maintained my mentor, the Aghori Vimalananda, "and women are creatures of emotion." In another version, "Women get technical about emotional things, and men get emotional about technical things." Sallie Tisdale has this to say: "It seems to me that men often move toward intimacy through sex, and women more often will move toward sex through intimacy. (That is, women are more afraid of the act of sex, and men of its consequences.)"

Male versus female?

Some believe that the sex-intimacy dichotomy may lie at the roots of human pair-bonding. Every mammal other than the human shows visible estrus (physical signs of fertility). Only we have lost our estrus, or our ability to distinguish it. Some biologists believe that one benefit of being able to disguise estrus is that it promotes monogamy, by encouraging a male to spend more of his time in the proximity of one female, copulating with her more frequently to ensure his paternity of her child. Another group is convinced that concealed estrus actually encourages a woman to mate with many men (on the sly, if need be). Since none of the men she mates with will be sure who is her child's father, all will be motivated to behave benignly toward the child.

The story of precisely why concealed estrus developed in humans is rather more complicated than such simplified arguments would lead us to believe. But whatever else this evolutionary adaptation may have accomplished, it has certainly made women (theoretically) sexually receptive almost all year round, and impaled men upon a paradox. Through this change men were given the opportunity to accomplish their ambition to gratify themselves continually, but they were simultaneously placed in peril by the possibility that their women might prove insatiably ungratifiable.

Couple sex with the magic and mystery inherent in menses, starring the vulva as a wound that heals itself and from which children miraculously emerge, and you have a situation in which many men began to see women as power objects that might be too powerful for their own good. Realizing that he (or she) who controls the means of production controls the product, men devised many ways to keep women under control. This happened in India as elsewhere, and many prominent Indian men of the past feared, or were at least uncomfortable with, the female creative power that Indians call shakti. Women being Nature's impulse to manifestation, the man who values manifestation will respect women as Nature's greatest boon, but the man who fears life will regard the female as the worst thing in the world. Many of India's priests still support a dogma which strictly separates sex from spirituality; to such men, women are the gateway to hell, both physically and mentally. Ironically, some of these men were sexoholics in early life (like St. Augustine), and when they renounced their indulgence they came to blame women (like St. Augustine) as the temptresses who had taught them to indulge.

Like our Western wedding rings, Indian wedding bangles and necklaces all symbolize the "tying down" of the bride's creativity to act within the confines of a specific context. Ideally, this channelling harnesses her energies effectively; all too often, though, women find themselves in the hands of pathologically inept men, who stifle that creativity. Fear of women has arisen from time to time in India, and many classical writings on the subject of women are depressingly sexist. But we should no more judge Ayurveda by such writings on the subject than we should judge all of American society on the writings of Pat Robertson, who has claimed that the passage of the equal-rights amendment would lead women to "leave their husbands, kill their children, practice witchcraft, destroy capitalism, and become lesbians."

Few men seem to realize that when they try to force women into positions of obedience they so impair the energies that flow through her that they often ruin what they hoped to perpetuate. Similarly, many women mistakenly think that hostile rebellion against male dominance is a remedy for the obstructions that that domination can produce. But demonizing men can be as injurious to the healthy flow of a woman's life force as being dominated by a man can be. Basically, we have no need for a society of fretful man-children and woman-children who are divided into hostile "feminist" and "men's movement" camps, continually tossing stones at one another.

Relationships

Healthy relationships are important to us all. Married people have lower death rates than single, widowed, or divorced people, and socially isolated individuals have well over twice the death rate of those who are socially connected, regardless of age, sex, or initial health status. Studies suggest that single people are at greater risk of arthritis, diabetes, peptic ulcers, back problems, gallstones, skin complaints, hypertension, varicose veins, breast cancer, stroke, prostate cancer, leukemia, heart disease, and migraines than are married people. Married couples and their children even had fewer fillings and better gums than did the members of divorced or bereaved families (whose grief, a vata-magnifying emotion, dries up their saliva). Married people are more likely to see a doctor sooner when they are ill, and to drink and smoke less heavily than divorced people.

Commitment counts, however; health benefits are stronger in those who are married than in those who merely cohabit. Quality of relationship also makes a difference, of course, and the same marital relationship that can provide health protection when it is healthy can create disease when it becomes dysfunctional. Routine marital disagreements can induce the fight or flight reaction, which releases the hormone cortisol into the circulation. When it remains briefly in the tissues, cortisol's presence is beneficial, but when it circulates too long in the organism it destroys the appetite, cripples the immune system, shuts down tissue repair, blocks sleep, and even breaks down bone. Women under stress show steeper cortisol rises that last longer than those in men, suggesting that they are much more sensitive to negative behavior than are men. A forty-year-old woman who is depressed (and so high in cortisol) may lose bone mass to the extent that she develops the bone density of a seventy-year-old woman.

Even when the relationship is healthy, wives tend to share their husbands' stresses. Strong links have been identified between a husband's occupation, his cause of death, and his wife's cause of death. Police sergeants and their wives both show high cancer rates, building laborers and their wives high rates of accidental death, doctors and their wives high suicide rates. Part of this is explainable by the fact that people tend to marry those with whom they share similar biological characteristics, right down to blood pressure. However, this is only part of the answer, because the same study found that a wife's career does not appear to have the same influence on her husband's cause of death.

It is difficult not to conclude that, knowingly or unknowingly, in their quest to preserve and protect their homes and families, women today often take on more emotional responsibilities than they can handle. As our relationships go, so our societies go, too, and our human civilization itself. If we are to begin to heal our relationships, we need first to begin healing ourselves. As our flows start to flow more healthily, our relationship with Nature will automatically resurrect itself. Then, if we listen to her, she can lead us in the directions that we need to go.

Sexual Communion

One of the ways to heal our relationships that she may suggest to us is healing through sexual communion. Sexual union is obviously not everything in life, but it is a vital part of a marriage, and men who search for ways to improve society really need look no further than their own sexual attitudes and practices. The *Charaka Samhita* clearly states that the best of all aphrodisiacs for a man is a woman who loves him: "All the delectable objects of the senses are found together in combination only in the person of the woman, nowhere else. . . . In her also are established righteousness, wealth, auspiciousness and the two worlds, this and the other."

But perfection of sexuality is founded not on improved technique, as many men seem to believe, but on transforming what is often a personal self-indulgence into a shared experience. The men of ancient India, who so appreciated the value of the "supreme aphrodisiac" that they intensively investigated a woman's sexual excitation and response, wrote down the results of their experiments in the sex manuals—the *Kama Sutra,* the *Ananga Ranga,* and the *Koka Shastra.* They correlate the lunar days with the female limb in which passion is automatically ignited on that day, and the means to awaken that passion. They outline sexual compatibility by the size and qualities of genitals, by personality, by homeland, and by astrology, palmistry, and physiognomy. They detail the varieties of enjoyment, including kissing, use of the nails, and Yoga postures as sexual positions, and provide recipes for alchemical aphrodisiacs, rejuvenatives, and remedies, and charms and spells for both men and women to attract the opposite sex.

These books, which opened broad new avenues of sexual pleasuring to the cognoscenti, did not, however, cause men to stop seeing sex as an indulgence. Many men, in fact, simply learned from them how to debauch more effectively. Ayurveda knew long ago what is now beginning to dawn on a few of us in the modern day: there is no point of satiation for food, sleep, or sex. No matter how much you eat today, your hunger will return tomorrow, even stronger than today's; the longer you sleep tonight, the longer you will want to sleep tomorrow night. And the more you indulge in the sort of sex that equals mutual masturbation, the more you will want of it, and the less you are likely to be pleased with it deep down inside where it counts.

The answer lies in realizing—not just intellectualizing, but coming to know with every cell of your body—that the partner with whom you unite is, for that moment that you are together, the embodiment of the universe in which you live. When you make love with someone you trust, you can learn to surrender, through him (or her), to Nature, and that surrender, if sincere, can do wonders for your flows. It can make your sex magical. If, for instance, a man were to honor his partner as the very embodiment of the goddess of wealth and prosperity, offering his seed into her would become an offering to that goddess, who would respond by sending prosperity to the couple.

What men first need to learn is how little they know of sex, and how much women can teach them. Men lack the neural connections that in a female integrate her groin with the upper portions of her brain, the connections that allow a higher form of consciousness to flow into her loins along with her lovemaking. Only a woman can train a man's nervous system to transcend its reptilian ancestry and mount toward a truly human response, for only a woman can teach a man to share her experience. Once both know how to share, the sky is the limit of the bliss they can generate and exchange together.

(NOTE: Sexual preference need not be an issue in enhancing

and spiritualizing your sexuality, although gay couples may find some difficulties in developing a consistent energy circuit between them because the "polarities" of their physical energies are identical.)

Doshas in Relationships

Physical compatibility is an important ingredient in sexual compatibility, which means that the doshas count for almost as much in your interpersonal relationships as they do in your relationship with Nature. Like doshas attract, and unlike doshas complement (when they do not repel). Once you decide on the sort of relationship you want to develop, you will know whether attraction or being complementary will be more important to it.

- Vata people require balance and relaxation. If they are already balanced and relaxed, two vata people can be the ideal stimulating company for one another; but if they are both out of balance and over-stimulated when they meet, two vatas will send one another over the edge.

- Pittas require a challenge, and if they have learned to pace their appetites, two pitta people might form an amazingly creative partnership. Two unbalanced pittas, however, will be Hitler and Mussolini to each other: both spouting and posturing, but the one always sullenly resenting that the other is the stronger, always in control.

- People of the kapha nature need motivation and stimulation. If they have both embarked on a program of healthy habits, two kaphas can find in one another the gentle reminders they need to stay on track. Two unreconstructed kaphas, however, will reinforce their mutual, natural tendencies to sloth, and mutually go to seed.

Pittas tend to rule a relationship; kaphas tend to submit, to promote harmony; vatas are unpredictable, sometimes submitting and sometimes seeking to be assertive. Mix two different people together, and their doshas will mix it up, vying for supremacy as doshas do within the confines of any living being. Most people are bi-doshic, of course, which makes the permutations all the more confusing and amusing: John's pitta is inflamed today after Mary's vata over-stimulated his kapha yesterday, and now he is trying to prevail upon her to renegotiate the agreement that her pitta got her a better deal on a few days back, when his kapha was projecting a spirit of compromise.

One way to approach this problem, which exists for everyone in every sort of relationship, is to pay close attention to your doshas and to the doshas of the people with whom you relate. Then you can learn how far you can go, in a certain context, before some negative influence kicks in your opposite number's imbalances and sends your relationship into a whirl.

Another way to relate is to keep referring your relationships back to Nature, and let her guide your actions, moment by moment. This allows you to ground yourself better in yourself, to find within some of the love and affection and validation that you require for balance. The more you can find within yourself, the less you will need to try to obtain from others. Soon you will find yourself so overflowing with harmony that you will begin to attract others to you, people who find that they feel a little better, a little calmer, when they sit in your presence. Then you are Nature's handmaiden, helping to change your corner of the world by channeling her sweetness into it.

Children

The people who most need you to be sweet for them, in every sense of that tasty word, are the ones who have appeared in the world through you. Their sweetness begins with yours, for childhood begins all the way back in the womb—or even further. When women who had been starved as fetuses during the first and second trimesters of their mothers' pregnancies during the Dutch Hunger Winter of 1944–45 delivered their own children, many of them were small, underweight infants. The grandmother's experience of privation had somehow affected the grandchildren. Ayurveda suggests, in fact, that a child is influenced by its ancestors as far back as the seventh previous generation. Like other, not necessarily pleasant realities of life, this may be a concern if your family health history, or that of your mate, displays some weaknesses. This warning flag should remind you that you will need to do whatever you can during your pregnancy to promote health in the little passenger within you, and that after the birth, your child may under certain circumstances need to be supplied with some extra healing energy.

It is also useful to remember that your baby has come to you with an inheritance of consciousness that will project itself through the platform that her heredity provides. Ayurveda, which generally supports the theory of reincarnation, suggests that souls select the situation into which they will be born. Children choose their parents—and in at least some cases it would appear that those who become children today were the parents, grandparents, or other previous relatives of the beings who become parents today. What goes around keeps coming back around, and it is wise to treat your fetus as if she possessed human awareness right from the moment of her conception, or even before.

Pregnancy

The ideal pregnancy begins six months or so before conception, when the two parents-to-be begin to purify and rejuvenate their bodies. When they feel in a state of optimal health they unite their seeds together, with joy and exaltation, at an auspicious moment. For the next nine months they should focus on welcoming their child-to-be into their family, for a child who spends "fetushood" in the aura of parents who do not want her will grow up feeling unwanted, no matter how much attention is lavished on the baby after her birth. Although the willful abortion of a fetus is not a desirable course of action for any of the parties involved, the lifelong scars created by an unwanted pregnancy may in some cases be worse that the physical and emotional trauma of a termination.

Once you have decided to bear your child, everything you eat and do and see and hear should be soft, pleasing, and wholesome, to reassure and strengthen the growing baby. "Like a pot brimful of oil," says the *Charaka Samhita,* "a pregnant woman should be handled without being upset in any way." Most women become somewhat "upset-prone" during pregnancy; for one thing, you are now not only eating for two, you are having to excrete for two, and the wastes of your fetus can clog your own channels. And, like any living being, the fetus also possesses doshas, and those extra doshas may kick your own into imbalance. Moreover, a woman's brain shrinks and her level of mental functioning decreases while she is pregnant, returning to normal only about six months after delivery. This is yet one more good reason to avoid work while you are pregnant and stay at home instead, quietly meditating, and bonding with the little soul who has come to live with you.

When an expectant mother becomes upset she also becomes upset for two, and strong sudden emotions, like the fear or anger that might be triggered by a frightening movie or television show, will affect your fetus more than it will affect you. The fetus can hear after the seventh month (some tiny babies can even recognize the theme songs from the soap operas their mothers watched during pregnancy!), but her emotions are awake from the very beginning. So, even though you may consider it an infringement of your personal freedom, make it a point to expose yourself only to wholesome influences while you are pregnant. Keep vigorous exercise, including sex, to a minimum during your pregnancy; replace it with a daily walk or a swim. Spend more of your time at home, particularly during and after the eighth month (which is when your body is busy transferring ojas to the baby), and make sure you do your socializing with people who love you. Your partner should facilitate these changes by spending extra time with you, helping to keep you comfortable and satisfied.

Deep-fried, very salty, or hot spicy food, large amounts of refined sugar, and the use of tobacco, alcohol, and caffeine are a few of the intakes that can disturb your guest. Sweet, bland, light food made from whole grains, fresh fruits, and vegetables is best. If you can digest milk, pregnancy is a very good time to drink a cup of warm milk with spices (saffron, cardamom, or ginger powder) to which you can add a half teaspoon of ghee and one to two teaspoons of raw honey. Weak ginger tea can help stave off nausea; so can eating a few pinches of roasted cumin or fennel seed, or sipping warm water with lemon and honey.

Ayurveda teaches that after the fetal heart begins to beat, mother and child begin to function as a "two-hearted" psychological unit. Some of the peculiar cravings that many pregnant women feel are due to a physical imbalance or a deficiency, or to the fetal wastes which strain her own waste-management systems. Most of these desires, though, reflect the fetus's own preferences, which influence the mother via the channels that connect them. It is good to satisfy such cravings, unless your health might be harmed by it. In addition, expectant mothers can consume a wide variety of Ayurvedically prepared tonics and supplements to promote the well-being of their two-hearted unit. Pregnant women should also nourish themselves by receiving regular prenatal massage, and in addition should massage themselves daily with a little oil (almond or olive oils are often most agreeable), paying special attention to nipples, abdomen, and vulva.

Childbirth

It is only since the 1960s that childbirth has come to be regarded as a medical condition. In the United States more babies are born (by induced labor) at 6 P.M. on Tuesdays than on any other day, for medical convenience; the fewest are born on Saturdays and Sundays. Since it is the fetal hormones that control onset of labor, medical convenience is likely to be quite disruptive to the delivery flow that the mother-child unit is ready to embark on. Further disruption can happen in the moments just after birth. The fetus begins her life and spends nine months of womb-time with the continual, rhythmic pulsation of her mother's heartbeat right above her. This makes it all the more important that a mother puts her baby to her left breast just after birth, so that she can hear this reassuring heartbeat during her first moments of extrauterine life.

This makes it imperative for an expectant mother to search carefully until she finds an obstetrician or midwife who appreciates her concerns, and a birthing location in which she feels relaxed and comfortable. She also needs to select a trusted labor companion, someone who can hold her hand lovingly, rub her back, remind her to breathe, and talk her through the whole process.

Ayurveda prefers that there be minimal interference with the birthing process, although some of its physicians use enemas of medicated oil to promote contractions by encouraging the free, strong, downward motion of vata, and give tonic herbs like saffron or ashvagandha to promote easy delivery. Then immediately after delivery, the mother is often given herbal decoctions to reduce her aches and pains and strengthen her nerves, and is later fed specially fortified foods to help her body regain its strength. In India, a newly delivered woman's well-oiled abdomen is gently bound with a cloth, to prevent the accumulation of vata in the now-empty womb.

At birth, the mother is introduced to the little being that she has carried and nourished for nine long months, and the baby is introduced to the world. In the section on childhood, we consider some of what it is most essential for the baby to receive during her first weeks and months of life (see pages 38–44). Now it is time to examine the child from her mother's point of view, and from the angle of the relationship between these two beings. No matter how old a child becomes, her mother remains her mother. Some mothers develop healthy relationships with their children during pregnancy itself, relationships that continue to widen and deepen as long as both are alive. Other mothers and children seem to be at odds from day one, and have to work very hard to maintain decent relations. The earlier in a child's life that a healthy relationship develops between the child and her mother, the healthier, calmer, and more contented that child will be, and will grow up to become.

Parenting

You cannot mandate or engineer a healthy relationship with your children. If it is to grow, it will grow in its own season, when it is watered with your love. Your best hope if you want your children to grow into healthy adults is to expose them to as many healthy habits as possible while they are young. As the Bible says, "Train up a child in the way he should go, and when he is old he will not depart from it."

Healthy Living

Follow a good Ayurvedic routine yourself, and if living that way seems to be doing good things for you, your child will automatically pick up parts of it herself. It is useless to try to force her to eat right, or sleep right, or live right; you can at best point her in that direction, and give her a good example to follow. Your baby ideally has one caregiver who is regularly available to her during the major part of the day for the first three years of her life. If at all possible, that caregiver should be the mother, for Nature has imbued mothers with a powerfully instinctual child-preserving consciousness that is protective in and of itself. And it is a great blessing to learn trust as a child, for you can then go through life trusting life.

As a parent, you have a tremendous responsibility to create this trust within your child, for the innocent sweetness of childhood dissipates all too soon, and the more of it your child can maintain, the more pleasant and satisfyingly youthful her later life will be. Your children are part of your own flow and part of your environment, and your health will be immeasurably better if your children are living healthy lives. It is sadly true, however, that it is not always possible in our current world for mothers to drop everything else they are doing and devote themselves to their children. Our society is rapidly returning to the old idea, "If you don't work, you don't eat." More than half the women in the United States who have children under the age of six are already working outside their homes or are looking for work, and more that half of all new mothers are working or looking for work within a year of the birth of a child. Reality counts: you can only do as much as you can. If you, as the baby's mother, cannot be its primary caregiver, see to it that you find enough assistance for yourself from other interested parties so that your baby never feels neglected or afflicted. If you must use day care, choose it carefully. Most, unfortunately, fail to provide the sort of constant role models a toddler requires; some children under the age of four in day care show high levels of cortisol (that stress hormone) when they are absent from their mothers for more than two hours at a time.

Whenever you do get time with your child, make use of her natural inquisitiveness to expose her to what you want her to learn. With some children you may be able to make dosha constitutionality a game, and show them how specific food, rest, exercise, meditation, and other practices affect different people in different ways. Others will refuse to cooperate with such foolishness. At all times, however, respect her intelligence, for if you are just using Ayurveda (or any other approach to health) as a means to some other end, she will quickly see through your game. The more hypocritical you are about overlooking your own indulgences while you pounce on hers, the less she will trust you. Above all, avoid unloading your own conflicts onto your child—she has not come into this world to parent you.

Learning and Supervision

As with food, so with every other aspect of life: introduce your baby to it slowly and gently, with your reassuring presence nearby. As she grows, expose her to a healthy way to live by living that way yourself. Ayurveda suggests that you indulge your baby in almost everything up to the age of three or four. The day she learns to say "no!" is a good day for you to start saying "no" to her. Set consistent, reasonable boundaries for her that are structured in love, and be as sweet and calm a disciplinarian as you can. Then allow her to make her own mistakes, while you watchfully do your best to prevent serious injury. This applies to anyone that it has fallen to your lot to parent: your own children, your step-children, your friend's children, your aged parents, perhaps even a sibling or two.

One good thing about a child's general kapha-predominance is that she is in many ways more resilient that an adult. Failure can be an excellent way for her to learn to succeed, as long as she fails gently enough, early enough in life. Allow your children to fail a little and don't fall into the trap of over-protecting them. You didn't learn to walk without falling flat on your face a few times. The sooner a child learns her own talents and her limits the better, particularly in this age of powerful peer pressure to conform to some "ideal." A child who begins to live too fast, burning away her innocence and sweetness, will age well before her time, and you as a parent should try to prevent this. If she learns from an early age the meaning of right and wrong, of healthy and poisonous, she is much less likely later to jump into danger on a whim even when her peers are pushing her to do so.

Children get up more enthusiastically after a fall when they know a parent is there to protect them, even when they know they'll be scolded for their foolhardiness. Be firm with your children, and when necessary, with pregnant women, the aged and the sick; but be nonviolent, in word and deed. Patience will, of course, be needed most at those moments when you are at the end of your rope and would cheerfully send the child off with the bogey man if only he would appear. But forbear, and keep forbearing, for violence begets violence. Studies show that children who bully others at school are themselves hit more often at home than are their peers, and their parents are more likely to approve of violent methods of problem-solving. Aggressive students also watch more violent television shows.

The most important thing for your "children" of any age, is that they feel safe, secure, and loved, and the best way to do that is to be there for them, literally. Very few kids who spend time each day at home with an adult end up bullying others; those who bully are usually the ones least supervised by adults. One of the real problems with the modern nuclear family is the lack of support, the amount of separation and "aloneness," that its members feel. One of the big benefits of India's extended or "joint" families is that when the mother is busy the baby can be cared for by big sister, auntie, grandma, or some cousin. Someone is always available to cuddle a child, to give her that human touch that is such a critical promoter of nutrition and immunity throughout life.

Immunization

Immunity is crucial, for it is often impossible to prevent your child from being exposed to the malevolent microorganisms that surround us. Many authorities today advise new parents to boost their children's immunity to disease through vaccination. If you are averse to immunizations, are confident that your child's resistance is always likely to be high, and have access to good medical knowledge and reliable remedies, you may be able to avoid vaccinations. But if your child's immunity is already somehow compromised, or if you live with her in a polluted environment that is swarming with microbes, immunization may be prudent. Even some physicians who distrust vaccination feel that all children should be immunized against polio and tetanus; although evidence also exists to suggest that HIV more readily infects the blood of people who have been inoculated with tetanus vaccine. There is no easy answer to the question of immunization, any more than there are easy answers to any of life's big questions. Each individual requires her own well-considered, carefully tailored program of health development, based on her own personal reality.

Storytelling

Bacteria and viruses are not the only pathogens in our environment. Even more beguiling parasites are the audio and video images of violence, sexual predation, bigotry, greed, and trivia with which the airwaves bombard us. Sitting young children down in front of the television is a particularly heinous form of "day care," both because it fills their minds with trash and because it retards the development of their brains. A child's mind becomes so habituated to images delivered in synch with sounds that its higher cortical structures never see any reason to develop. In the words of humanitarian author Joseph

Chilton Pearce, television "provides a synthetic counterfeit of what the brain itself is supposed to produce in response to language, as in storytelling." Habituation to television may even prevent the further development of the higher brain structures needed to create internal imagery.

One of the best ways to erect these essential brain structures in your child is to tell her a story. Each new story challenges the young brain and mind to develop a whole new set of neural connections, which creates an appetite for more. One of the greatest losses we have experienced as a culture is the loss of the "grandmother tales" that our parents and grandparents used to use to develop the young minds of their offspring. Storytelling is the ideal form of vaccination against the putrid semblances of reality that pass for popular culture, the best guarantee against invasion by "techno-ama."

Tell your children stories as they grow; help them to think, visualize, evolve. Introduce them to as many images of healthy living as you can, for what they see they will become. Take tales from literature, make them up, borrow them from friends. Transmit the family history, warts and all, to your offspring; let them see that people can learn to love and care for one another, even amid life's imperfections.

Vow Stories: Vrata Katha

Once upon a time, human culture was transmitted from one generation to the next through such storytelling. Grandparents and parents would impart the tales and myths of their societies to wide-eyed children, creating thereby a link between the culture's past and its future. Sadly, in modern societies myth has become so equated with fiction, and we have become so convinced that the new is always superior to the old, that we have jettisoned most of our ancient, tried-and-true mythic realities.

Instead, we search vainly for new narratives and new mores upon which to build our brave new worlds. People cannot do without myths, and if they have lost their own they will manufacture new ones. Whether this involves revering with a near-religious sanctity one's homeland, favorite movie star, sports team, or religious cult, a sizeable proportion of our population has taken on images that are merely the addictive drugs of the mythic world. Worse, we are raising a generation who has no positive images to lose—a generation who knows no world other than that presented by television and the Internet. We have lost touch with Nature, and gone "virtual." Billions today live for nothing more noble in life than their own indulgence, spurred into ever-increasing self-gratification by the "consumption is happiness" fiction.

As our families have fragmented, we have been losing that current of affinity that provides continuity in our societies. We are pulling our culture up by its roots and gaily tossing it onto the fire of our promiscuous self-indulgence. When life's focus shifts from "us" to "me," that flow between the generations that make up a family, and between the people who make up a community, is cut off. All the energy gets so dammed up inside "me" that none remains to nourish "thee." But how can I hope to maintain a healthy flow within myself for very long if my every act impedes healthy flow between myself and my environment?

The situation is grave, but it is not yet hopeless. Wise use of the valuable traditions we have inherited from our forebears can still provide our children with healthy images. The older ones among us are ideally positioned to devote some of their retired lives to the telling of noble, meaningful stories to children. Anyone who adopts this simple course of action can be confident that she is truly doing her bit to ensure that our civilization will continue to flow along, to irrigate the generations that will come after us.

Spiritual Development

Storytelling can also serve as one path to spiritual development. In India, women have taken a whole class of specialized myth stories of gods, goddesses, magical beings, heroes, and saints for ritual use. While the ancient Vedic ritual is monopolized by men, the spiritual tradition of women is one of the vow *(vrata)*. Vows can be annual, monthly, or specially scheduled when a woman has a desire to be fulfilled. Most vows follow a similar pattern: after first purifying yourself you fast for a day (occasionally two), alone or in the company of other women, praying, singing and chanting, and telling these "vow stories" *(vrata katha)*. Your vow becomes complete when, after your final worship ritual, you distribute consecrated food to all and then break your own fast.

Vows create compacts between women and Nature. In the past they have most often been aimed at attracting a healthy, loving spouse, preserving that spouse's health and welfare, gaining children, solving problems, receiving inspiration, or obtaining an answer for a pressing question. There is no reason, however, why they could not be directed to other objects, including the getting or keeping of a job. "What you envision, you become," says an ancient proverb. If you envision health, happiness, and prosperity for your family, those things will surely develop—eventually. How swiftly or gradually they develop will depend (among other things) on your level of determination, and on the obstacles that lie in your way.

Removing obstacles caused by adverse astral influences has been, and remains, one of the most common reasons that women make and keep vows. Such practices are connected with the several Indian systems of astrology which are known collectively as *Jyotish*. A good example of one of these vow stories is for the planet Saturn; it is now available in English translation with commentary (by the author of this book) as *The Greatness of Saturn* (see bibliography).

A vow need not be Indian to work for you. Vows are also part of the Christian, Muslim, Buddhist, and Jain traditions, among others, and there is nothing standing in the way of your taking any myth and creating a vow for it. Find a story that is meaningful and important to you, one that you would like to have in your own life, and develop a relationship with it. Be patient, be consistent and maternal; nourish it like you would a small child, and then see what happens. If it likes you it will come to live with you, and you will have gained a precious gift to pass on to your own flesh and blood.

Life is relationship, and no life or relationship is flawless. No matter how hopeless a relationship may seem, despairing over it is not likely to help. If you have drawn your last straw, take off a day to fast, observe a vow, and relieve the pressure by taking your problem to Nature, who is always there to lend you a listening ear. All Nature asks of you is that you do your best to live your life as well as you can, to do what is most appropriate and wholesome for yourself, your family, your country, and the world. Try to live your life in such a way that at the end of each day you have done what you could, however insignificant that may sometimes seem to you, and you will ensure for yourself a life whose flavor is sweet.

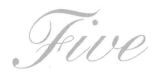

THE WISE WOMAN

THE VATA AGE

The principles of life do not change when you graduate into older age. Life is still relationship; your relationship with yourself still forms the basis of your relationship with any other being; and you remain a body-mind-spirit complex. But now the focus of your existence shifts to the spirit. Childhood was your window for optimum development of your body, and adulthood your opportunity to maximize your mind. With your senior years comes the precious chance to extend your consciousness from the matter of the body-mind, with all its limitations, into the less restricted consciousness of the spirit. This does not mean that you should turn all your flows inward and withdraw from society; on the contrary, since vata likes to spread and to expand, the vata time of your life is a fine opportunity to disseminate your experiences to others. What you should be withdrawing from is the self-absorption you had, first during your kapha-structured formative years and then during your busy, pitta-dominated full-grown years. Kapha people will still require motivation and stimulation, pittas will still appreciate a challenge, and vata types will still do best with balance and relaxation. But your dedication to your own self-importance, that is, in your constitution as well as in your physical-mental-emotional-spiritual condition, should be ready to wane.

After menopause, both body and mind deteriorate, gradually, if you have lived well until then, and more quickly if you have not. Like it or not, you are headed for the terminal phase of your existence: your death. When you are born, you can be certain about one thing, and one thing only, and that is that one day you are, without any doubt, going to die. You may postpone the inevitable by living right and taking supplements, but no pill or activity has yet been found that is guaranteed to make you immortal. If you have a heartfelt reason to live, that may be enough of a spur to keep you going long after your time should have been up—but even that reprieve is temporary.

Mentors and gurus from time immemorial have taught that to know life, you must study death. According to Indian tradition, the postmenopausal years are a fine time for an individual (or couple) to move into this, the "forest-dwelling" *(vanaprastha)* phase of existence. In the past, this meant leaving the big house, which is filled with the hustle and bustle of the joint family, and moving to a small (but quite comfortable) hut in the forest, neither too far from, nor too near your previous home. There in the hut you go about your daily routine, which has by now become second nature to you, and in your ample spare time you have occasion to reflect. As you look back over your life, you compare and contrast it with the lives of your peers, and the lives of past generations. As these memories jostle and juxtapose within you, a layer of wisdom gradually rises to the top of your churning awareness, a wisdom that deepens and enriches the flavor of your life's sweetness.

Grandparenting

The children whose lives you had supervised are now on their own, with children of their own. And your role in their lives metamorphoses from parent to mentor as your children come to realize the value of the wisdom implicit in your advice, and as your children's children come to you to be grandparented. "Grandchildren are the reward you get for having children," says one of my friends, who became a first-time grandmother in her late forties. Graduating to grandmotherhood permits you to do grandmotherly things with your grandchildren: bake them pies, tell them stories, take them on walks and adventures, pamper, love, instruct, spoil, and otherwise do things to enrich their lives that their parents may not have the time or the inclination to do for them.

I still remember my mother's father for the childlike affection with which he used to take the younger versions of me and my sister to his town's soda fountain to buy each of us a lemonade. It was something we could look forward to each day that we stayed there over the holidays, a certainty that we counted on for many years. We also came to count on some excitement awaiting us with our grandmother when we returned from our excursion into town. Maybe she would take us out with her to feed the chickens, or let us help her bake the biscuits, or show us the catalogs for the cosmetics that she sold.

Our father's parents lived just a few houses away and we made regular pilgrimages there, too, to the garden whose cucumbers and cabbages would become mouth-watering pickles and sauerkraut, to the pecan trees whose nuts would be transmuted into pecan squares in our grandma's oven. Inside the house we would eat those squares and kolaches and other Czech pastries while we watched our granddad whittle and contrive and repair. Once he took me with him to help him bolt up the sideboards on a (what seemed gargantuan to me then) livestock transport truck. I remember that day vividly, even now: the oily film of lubricant on the black steel bolts, the sudden evergreen fragrance released as the washers bit into the wood, the bonhomie of working alongside my granddad, man to man.

What children look for in grandparents is memories of being loved by them without expectations or restrictions. This is what makes grandparents such a crucial ingredient in the family recipe. My sister and I have been immensely lucky in this way, for even today our family ties are strong. It does help that most of our relatives still live in or near that small town, but it is by no means essential that your family be composed of blood relatives. Your "family" members, as Barbara Kingsolver put it, are "the people you won't let go of for anything," and you may well find them far beyond the ranks of your kin. The woman who became my parents' "second daughter" began life as my sister's best friend during her years in secondary school; my own mentor's foster daughter has herself now gained "associate status" in our family. Where you find your family is less important than what you do with them.

Menopause

After menopause, a woman should be sufficiently experienced in life to begin to coach the family team, to mentor the younger women in it by offering advice and encouragement, teaching them her own rituals and vow stories, and generally setting a good example for them. It is, of course, much easier to be a good mentor and a good example if you are healthy, and many women today remain hale and hearty long after their male contemporaries have bitten the dust.

But modern medicine has been trying to work the same "magic" on menopause that it has been working on childbirth, to convert what is a normal life transition into a "medical event" or, worse yet, a "disease." Fortunately, other scientists are working against them, discovering evidence as to why menopause may be essential to humankind. Menopause began, apparently, when evolution increased the size of the human head to enable it to accept the larger human brain. Human babies are less developed than other species at birth, at least in part, because if their heads were allowed to grow to full size in the womb they would be unable to get through the human birth canal. Babies must therefore remain helplessly dependent on their mothers for years after they are born.

In the past, as women aged they probably carried on delivering children, as well as having to continue to care for the older ones as well. But the likelihood of dying as a result of pregnancy or labor increases for a woman as she ages, as do the chances of her new infant failing to thrive or survive. If she does die, she endangers the survival of her existing children, whose chances improve if she stops having children while she is still relatively healthy and vital. As Dr. Jared Diamond explains: "In effect, the older mother is risking more for less potential gain. That is one set of factors that would tend to favor human female menopause and that would paradoxically result in a woman having more surviving children by giving birth to fewer children." In addition, an older woman who is no longer preoccupied with the requirements of pregnancy and lactation can assist others with delivery and mother and baby care, she can babysit and direct the education of the young ones, and can forage for food for the family. In this way, she supports both the propagation of her own genetic material and the evolution of humanity as a whole. Menopause also serves her personal evolution, for as age advances, ojas retreats. When it no longer contains sufficient ojas to contribute to the production of a new life, a woman's body shuts down its reproductive capabilities, and redirects its ojas to other projects.

Crisis?

Most of us equate menopause with its final sense of "cessation of menstruation," which happens at roughly the same age all around the world (about fifty-one, though about 10 percent of women reach menopause before the age of forty). Actually, though, menopause is a process that begins between the ages of thirty and thirty-five as the body crests at its fittest, healthiest, and juiciest point. In those societies where age is valued over youth, a woman is seen as coming into her own at menopause, and so is likely to have less problems with the transition. Where youth is emphasized, as in the West, the opposite is the case, and she is likely to perceive herself as being on the slippery slope of a steep and terrible decline. None of the Indian women I know who live a predominantly traditional life have ever complained to me of menopausal symptoms (they have complained about lots else, though!); the women that I know in India who have mentioned hot flashes, insomnia, and mood changes are those who have become Westernized in their outlook and habits.

Just because they don't complain doesn't mean that they don't suffer, of course, but even so, menopause is clearly not the crisis in India that it has been portrayed in the West. Nor does it seem to be in many other Asian societies; the Japanese language, for example, has no word for "hot flashes." And menopause does not affect every Western woman in the same way: my own mother reported that she just stopped bleeding one day, and that was that. Seventy-five percent of American women, however, experience at least some hot flashes, night sweats, and vaginal dryness. Twenty percent (on average) experience hot flashes for less than a year, but 25 to 50 percent struggle with them for more than five years.

Symptoms

Some of the other common "symptoms" of menopause are drying out and thinning of the skin, thinning hair, insomnia, migraines, anxiety, depression, mood swings, mental fogginess, and short-term memory loss. All these are characteristic of disturbed vata. Vata, which is bound to increase as you move into the vata phase of your life, increases even more at menopause because this is a transition period, a "joint." As we have discovered, vata always increases at joints, and it tends to become particularly perturbed in conditions of strong disparity.

Even hot flashes, although they are hot, are primarily manifestations of this quality of disparity that becomes prominent due to the vata imbalance. If pitta has accumulated over many years the hot flashes are likely to be more frequent, more intense, and more irritating, and your mood is likely to be more irritable. Kapha derangement during this passage may also contribute a symptom or two of its own (such as weight gain or fluid retention). But vata remains the mistress of this particular bodily ceremony, and this is the reason why something as simple as deep breathing (performed on its own or in combination with yoga and with meditation) can reduce or even eliminate hot flashes in some afflicted women.

Disparity explains why women whose bodies have grown habituated to high levels of estrogen are more likely to suffer menopausal symptoms. "Ample estrogen" states can develop insidiously: for example, when a woman whose liver is not metabolizing estrogen effectively consumes a diet that is high in cholesterol. When "high-level estrogen" women enter menopause, they are forced to come off that addiction "cold turkey." One positive effect of lowering ambient estrogen levels is that the symptoms of fibroids and endometriosis that many estrogen-addicted women display usually decline with the decline in estrogen. But the potential negatives of coming off an estrogen addiction can be severe: these include increased serum cholesterol, heart disease, and osteoporosis.

Osteoporosis

Your bone density peaks at around the age of thirty-five, and then begins to decline. If you have built it up carefully before that age, and take care of yourself thereafter, it will coast its way down. If you did not work to build it up while you were young, and do not work to retain it as you grow old, it will plummet below the fracture level, causing bones like your hip to fracture spontaneously. Whether you will age gracefully and healthily or not will depend on how you live your daily life before you reach the threshold of old age. Quick medical fixes are no substitute for the regular daily performance of health-building routines that empower the organism to refuse to fall ill.

If you are willing to work with your body, and with Nature, you can swim your way through menopause. You will need to continue to exercise and eat healthily, but if good habits are making you feel good, why would you want to stop them? You may gain a little weight, but a small increase in your fat stores during menopause may actually be beneficial. Added heaviness can help to ballast vata's erratic tendencies, and the extra fat will facilitate production of your own internal estrogen. Becoming vegetarian may be helpful: vegetarians need less calcium than do meat-eaters (when proteins are digested, the body uses up calcium to remove their wastes). You may want to increase your intake of foods like garlic (provided your pitta is not too high), which promotes bone health, and tofu, which exerts an estrogenic effect once it is inside you.

You will have to keep a watchful eye on pitta: too low, and your

RISK FACTORS

Osteoporosis is predominantly a disease of women (the ratio of women to men it affects is 3:1 or more). Some of the risk factors for osteoporosis are:

- Having missed many menstrual periods during your fertile life
- Menopause before the age of 45
- White skin (Asians come second)
- Insufficient body fat
- Family history of osteoporosis
- Poor diet, especially a diet high in animal protein, sodium, and white sugar, and low in potassium
- Smoking, drinking, carbonated drinks, and other pitta-increasing factors
- History of insufficient weight-bearing exercise
- Long-term use of certain medications (including steroids, thyroid hormone, and some chemotherapeutic agents)

digestion will suffer; too high, and your hot flashes may increase. Pitta's acidity has been implicated in osteoporosis: one study showed that postmenopausal osteoporosis was reduced in women who consumed the antacid potassium bicarbonate in amounts that neutralized the excess acid in their systems. This was probably due partly to the antacid and partly to the potassium, for excessive antacid use can lower stomach acid, which may actually impede calcium absorption.

It is never too late to get some benefit from changing your diet and habits, and ideally these changes will stimulate the body itself to do what it needs to do: to produce more hormone, preserve its skin, and reallocate its ojas. But if you have waited until menopause to begin to put your physical affairs in order, you may find your bone density decreasing despite all your best efforts to take calcium and exercise. During the years in which your body is adjusting to the loss of its estrogen addiction, vata causes your bone mass to decrease faster, and some women lose as much as 20 percent of the total mass of their bones.

Hormone Replacement

If you know that you are at risk of osteoporosis, or if hot flashes or other symptoms torment you stubbornly, you may need to replace your diminishing hormones.

Sometimes phytohormones (which are derived from plants) suffice. Some women find that progesterone alone (derived from wild yam) works well; others also add soy- or licorice-derived estrogens. Phytoestrogens are also found in clover, alfalfa, flax seed, and other plants. Some of these have been reported to exert toxic effects on the reproductive organs, and so must be used with care.

Paradoxically, phytoestrogens may also have a partial anti-estrogen effect, because they compete with the body's natural estrogen for its estrogenic receptors. This means that some of these substances may be able to help prevent heart disease and osteoporosis, while they prevent the recurrence of breast cancer. It is not unreasonable to think that phytoestrogens might also act to help prevent breast cancer from developing in high-risk women. If it transpires that phytoestrogens can be used in this way, it is also likely that they will produce fewer side effects than does tamoxifen.

Phytohormones do not, however, work as well for all women as does hormone replacement therapy (HRT), and in this matter it is wise for a woman to work carefully with her doctor. Administered under the care of a well-trained physician, HRT can be safe and effective—when used for the right reasons. But it is unhealthy to do as an increasing number of women are doing and take HRT simply to try to stay young—in effect this is maintaining an estrogen addiction because you are afraid of the consequences to your appearance should you give it up. Taking HRT for cosmetic reasons denies your tissues the opportunity to age gracefully, and prevents your mind from being able to mature into its second (after childhood), and potentially longer-lasting, low-hormone stage of life.

Rejuvenation

Fundamentally, though, the problem is not an excess of this or a lack of that, nor is the full answer to it one of reducing one thing and increasing another. The answer is rejuvenation, *rasayana*, "the path of juice." Aging means loss of life's "juice," literally as well as figuratively. Bodies shrink with age, minds turn woozier. Joints dry out and leak; muscles lose tone. The aged even feel cold more acutely than do the young, as vata dessicates their insulating body fat. Paying close attention to your "state" becomes particularly important during your vata years. For when you are feeling not quite right and do nothing about it, a "pre-disease" situation can snowball into an illness far more quickly than it might have done in your earlier years. Couple this tendency with the greater likelihood of degenerative diseases like arthritis, and you can go downhill quickly if you neglect your being.

Rejuvenation with substances is now quite essential to shore up declining vitality. Small amounts of several substances should be consumed regularly, in particular preparations such as chyvanaprasha, which are basically medicated foods. Regular skin care is also essential, less for vanity than because vata is specially connected to the sense of touch, and so to the skin. Keeping your skin well oiled is one of the most reliable ways to keep vata under control. Now is a good time to make regular pilgrimages to your masseuse, especially if she has learned some of Ayurveda's specialized oil-application techniques such as *pizhichil* and *dhara*.

Pizhichil (known in Sanskrit as *kaya seka* or *sarvanga dhara*) involves the application, for over an hour or more, of heated medicated oil to all limbs of the body. Two or four helpers squeeze the oil onto the body from cloth sponges from a height of several inches and gently massage it over the skin. Dhara (more properly, *shiro dhara*) is the pouring of a liquid (usually medicated oil, milk, or buttermilk) onto the forehead from a height of about 3 inches. This is performed for half an hour to an hour and a half daily, usually in the morning, after first oiling the head and body.

A Purposeful Life

Rasayana returns to you some of the life juice that you lost as your organism aged. From the physical angle, HRT is a sort of rasayana, since it replenishes your "hormone juices." But physical vitality is not all there is to youthfulness. Rejuvenation really implies a return to the natural kind of sweetness that a child possesses. Maybe you missed a happy childhood; maybe your midlife was filled with crisis. However, you can overcome any lingering bitterness that is corroding you inside if you are willing to forgive.

Ayurveda's word for immunity, *vyadhikshamatva*, literally means "forgiveness of disease." Dredging up the past again and again to verbalize ancient grievances anew simply inflates a problem that can be solved only by releasing it from your being. When you are willing to let bygones be bygones, when you can release yourself from the jail you have created of your own memories, you will give your spirit the kind of breathing room it requires to flourish. Then, when it bears fruit, you can taste a juice that is permanent, and one whose sweetness will never go stale. Ayurveda promotes physical rejuvenation, not to facilitate the running of marathons at the age of ninety-five, but to assist the body and mind to retain enough of their vigor in order that they will not interfere with the spiritual development that is your proper pastime as you age.

"Life extension" is now a fad, with some researchers talking of eventually pushing the human life span to 400 years. But even if rasayanas of both varieties could give you an extra century or two of life, how useful would it be if you had nothing in particular to live for? What kind of life is it that has no purpose behind it? It is no wonder that a large percentage of retirees (men especially) fall prey to serious ailments shortly after they retire. Each day has an empty hole (vata) in it where work used to be, when you retire without any clue about what to do with your retired self.

If you want to live healthily you have to live purposefully, as my parents do. They exercise daily; my father single-handedly tends his mammoth garden. They stimulate their minds a bit each day with the help of books and crossword puzzles. They eat right, after seeing how well it made them feel (my insistence that they experiment dietetically may have encouraged them somewhat in this). They distribute their mountains of surplus home-grown food to their friends and neighbors, and try always to be alert to the needs of others who may be reluctant to ask for their assistance.

The Importance of Prayer

My parents are no more perfect than any other human beings, which is to say that they fall prey to irrationality at times, argue about trifles, and fail to live up to their own expectations. But they are far healthier, in both mind and body, than many of their peers because they are healthier in spirit. They act on their religious beliefs by serving others, studying the Bible, and (above all) by praying. Prayer changes things; the act of sitting quietly with God allows God into your inner being, where transformations are waiting to occur. If you have lost the threads of your life's purpose, you can find them again through prayer. If you have forgotten how to pray, or you were never taught when you were younger, there is still time! Go out and find a mentor, a wise man or woman whose own purpose can infect you with the determination to live in states of consciousness that are higher and finer than the ones in which most of us usually exist. If you are genuinely sincere, your search will eventually introduce you to that divinely permanent and invincible order (in Sanskrit, *ritam*) that is the source of all our more limited and temporary human harmonies.

The day that spiritual harmony dawns on your horizon you will find yourself ready to take responsibility for any imbalance in your environment, and to contribute in whatever way you can to improve what needs to be improved around you. As you let go of the idea that you can teach others you will realize that, like you, others can learn what health really means. When you learn how to change yourself, your example automatically begins to show other people how to change themselves. Our violent medical system is a reflection of our violent society; the beginning of forgiveness, however halting and imperfect, is the beginning of the end of brutality.

Death

Recognition of the oneness of life often signals the beginning of the end of individual existence, too. What better death can you have, than to die when you are at your healthiest? It may sound paradoxical, but if we use the contemporary American writer Thomas Moore's phrase, "paradox is usually a sign of the presence of soul."

Awareness of the inevitability of death is something that everyone should learn young. It was easy to do so in the past, when death was all around us; children saw death on a daily basis, and though they may never have learned to love it they at least learned to accept it. But today we who are afraid of death have put it out of sight, so that we may forget about it until it is upon us. How foolish we are, residents of a world in which situations can change in a heartbeat, when any moment could be our last, to believe that somehow death will not come for us!

Birth to childhood to adulthood to procreation to decline and death—this is the cycle of life's eternal regenerating and releasing dynamism of embodied consciousness. How will you know its rhythm in full if you try to exclude its culmination? My mentor had me take death as my adviser. He told me to keep asking myself, "If death were to come for me right now, right this moment, would I be ready for it? Is what I am doing at this moment worthy of being the final act of my life? If not, make it so!"

The final relationship of your life is your relationship with death. If you are able to stay centered and to embrace death wholeheartedly, if you have made yourself ready for death by the time that death is ready for you, then yours will be a life that is well lived, a life whose last memory will be one of the infinite bounty of Nature's sweetness.

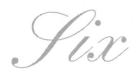

NATURE

THE AGELESS ONE

Birth to death to birth again, again, and again, over and over, for hundreds of generations, until we come to where we sit today, at a truly critical moment in the history of the human race. Will we continue slouching toward a materialist, consumer-friendly, mass-market utopia, unthinkingly poisoning ourselves into oblivion, or will enough of us wake up in time to steer our families and communities back in the direction of a sustainable civilization? I am confident that Nature will not allow us to destroy ourselves, although I fear that she may feel the need to rough us up a bit so that we become willing to start seeing things her way again.

Each of us must do what we can to assist Nature in this work, and for many of us the best we can do will be to do what we can to keep our little corners of the world healthy and harmonious. Every act of compassion has the potential to produce far-ranging effects, and to help even one person to become healthier and happier is to do the same, on a smaller scale, for Nature. As you go about your daily work, if you try to keep this broader perspective in mind, it is bound to make your day move more smoothly. When you interact with someone you do not care for, or take up some work that you hate to do, your task will become that much easier if you offer your efforts to Nature, and try to see things from her perspective.

And when you start to see things from Nature's perspective, you are likely to find compassion for her arising in your heart. How hard she works for us, and how much we abuse her! Even Nature is bound to feel weary of all her responsibilities, from time to time, and it is at those moments that she can use some support. She doesn't require much; even a kind word or a friendly gesture is enough to overjoy her. Nature is pleased when a child innocently garlands a tree or decorates a stone. Whenever an older woman takes a younger woman in hand, to offer the benefit of her years of experience, Nature smiles. Your monthly blood is the seal on the covenant that Mother Nature has made with you, and when you put aside a few moments during your bleeding time consciously to renew your bond with her, it satisfies her immensely.

As you navigate your way down your life's river, through childhood and adulthood and old age, always try to keep your eye on Nature. Make her your mentor and adviser, your friend and confidante, let her guide you on your path, and you will never find any impediment to your flow that you will not be able to overcome. Confidence begets confidence; so rely on her, and wherever you roam you will always feel right at home. Keep your relationship with Nature in good repair, and you will find your life blossoming in ways you never dreamed possible. Take care of Nature and she will, without the least doubt, always keep you in the palm of her hand.

Appendix 1

FOOD GUIDELINES
FOR BASIC
CONSTITUTIONAL TYPES

The guidelines provided in the tables that follow are general, giving foods that influence the doshas. Specific adjustments may need to be made for individual requirements (for example, for food allergies, strength of agni, season of the year, and degree of dosha predominance or aggravation). **No** means that the foods aggravate or increase the dosha. Avoid eating these if you are following a diet that pacifies the dosha. **Yes** means that the foods pacify or decrease the dosha. Select food from this column if you are following a diet that pacifies the dosha.

FRUIT				*ok in moderation **ok rarely	
VATA		**PITTA**		**KAPHA**	
No	**Yes**	**No**	**Yes**	**No**	**Yes**
Generally most dried fruit	*Generally most sweet fruit*	*Generally most sour fruit*	*Generally most sweet fruit*	*Generally most sweet & sour fruit*	*Generally most astringent fruit*
Apples (raw)	Apples	Apples (sour)	Apples	Avocados	Apples
Cranberries	(cooked)	Apricots	(sweet)	Bananas	Applesauce
Dates (dry)	Applesauce	(sour)	Apple sauce	Coconuts	Apricots
Figs (dry)	Apricots	Bananas	Apricots	Dates	Berries
Pears	Avocados	Berries	(sweet)	Figs (fresh)	Cherries
Persimmons	Bananas	(sour)	Avocados	Grapefruit	Cranberries
Pomegranates	Berries	Cherries	Berries	Kiwi fruit	Figs (dry)*
Prunes (dry)	Cherries	(sour)	(sweet)	Mangoes**	Grapes*
Raisins (dry)	Coconuts	Cranberries	Cherries	Melons	Lemons*
Watermelons	Dates (fresh)	Grapefruit	(sweet)	Oranges	Limes*
	Figs (fresh)	Grapes	Coconuts	Papayas	Peaches
	Grapefruit	(green)	Dates	Pineapples	Pears
	Grapes	Kiwi fruit**	Figs	Plums	Persimmons
	Kiwi fruit	Lemons	Grapes (red	Rhubarb	Pomegranates
	Lemons	Mangoes	& purple)	Tamarinds	Prunes
	Limes	(green)	Limes*	Watermelons	Raisins
	Mangoes	Oranges	Mangoes		Strawberries*
	Melons	(sour)	(ripe)		
	Oranges	Peaches	Melons		
	Papayas	Persimmons	Oranges		
	Peaches	Pineapples	(sweet)		
	Pineapples	(sour)	Papayas*		
	Plums	Plums (sour)	Pears		
	Prunes	Rhubarb	Pineapples		
	(soaked)	Strawberries	(sweet)		
	Raisins	Tamarinds	Plums		
	(soaked)		(sweet)		
	Rhubarb		Pomegranates		
	Strawberries		Prunes		
	Tamarinds		Raisins		
			Watermelons		

VEGETABLES				*ok in moderation **ok rarely	
VATA		PITTA		KAPHA	
No	Yes	No	Yes	No	Yes
Generally frozen, raw, & dried	*Generally cooked*	*Generally pungent*	*Generally sweet & bitter*	*Generally sweet, juicy, & bitter*	*Generally most pungent*
Artichoke	Asparagus	Eggplant**	Artichoke	Zucchini	Artichoke
Eggplant	Beet	Beet (raw)	Asparagus	Cucumber	Asparagus
Beet greens*	Cabbage*	Beet greens	Beet (cooked)	Olives (black	Eggplant
Bitter melon	(cooked)	Burdock root	Bitter melon	& green)	Beet
Broccoli	Carrots	Daikon radish	Broccoli	Parsnips**	Beet greens
Brussels	Cauliflower*	Garlic	Brussels sprouts	Pumpkin	Bitter melon
sprouts	Coriander	Green chilis	Cabbage	Squash (winter)	Broccoli
Burdock root	Zucchini	Horseradish	Carrots (cooked)	Sweet potato	Brussels sprouts
Cabbage (raw)	Cucumber	Kohlrabi**	Carrots (raw)*	Taro root	Burdock root
Cauliflower	Daikon radish*	Leeks (raw)	Cauliflower	Tomatoes (raw)	Cabbage
(raw)	Fennel (anise)	Mustard greens	Celery		Carrots
Celery	Garlic	Olives (green)	Coriander		Cauliflower
Dandelion	Green beans	Onions (raw)	Zucchini		Celery
greens	Green chilis	Peppers (hot)	Cucumber		Coriander
Horseradish**	Jerusalem	Prickly pear	Dandelion		Daikon radish
Kale	artichokes*	(fruit)	greens		Dandelion greens
Kohlrabi	Leafy greens*	Radishes (raw)	Fennel (anise)		Fennel (anise)
Mushrooms	Leeks	Spinach	Green beans		Garlic
Olives (green)	Lettuce*	(cooked)**	Jerusalem		Green beans
Onions (raw)	Mustard greens*	Spinach (raw)	artichokes		Green chilis
Peas (raw)	Okra	Sweet corn	Kale		Horseradish
Peppers (sweet	Olives (black)	(fresh)**	Leafy greens		Jerusalem
& hot)	Onions	Tomato	Leeks (cooked)		artichokes
Potatoes	(cooked)*	Turnip greens	Lettuce		Kale
Prickly pear	Parsley*	Turnips	Mushrooms		Kohlrabi
(fruit & leaves)	Parsnip		Okra		Leafy greens
Radishes (raw)	Peas (cooked)		Olives (black)		Leeks
Sweet corn	Pumpkin		Onions (cooked)		Lettuce
(fresh)**	Radishes		Parsley		Mushrooms
Tomato	(cooked)*		Parsnips		Mustard greens
(cooked)**	Spaghetti		Peas		Okra
Tomato (raw)	squash*		Peppers (sweet)		Onions
Turnips	Spinach (raw		Potatoes		Parsley
Wheat grass	& cooked)*		Prickly pear		Peas
sprouts	Sprouts*		(leaves)		Peppers (sweet
	Squash		Pumpkin		& hot)
	(summer &		Radishes		Potatoes
	winter)		(cooked)		Prickly pear
	Rutabaga		Spaghetti		(fruit & leaves)
	Sweet potato		squash		Radishes
	Taro root		Sprouts (not		Rutabaga
	Turnip greens*		spicy)		Spaghetti squash*
	Watercress		Squash (summer		Spinach
			& winter)		Sprouts
			Rutabaga		Summer squash
			Sweet potato		Sweet corn
			Taro root		Tomato (cooked)
			Watercress*		Turnip greens
			Wheat grass		Turnips
			sprouts		Watercress
					Wheat grass
					sprouts

N.B.: Always use suitable grains when "generic" items are given	GRAINS		*ok in moderation **ok rarely		

VATA		PITTA		KAPHA	
No	Yes	No	Yes	No	Yes
Barley	Amaranth*	Bread (with	Amaranth	Bread (with	Amaranth*
Bread (with	Durum flour	yeast)	Barley	yeast)	Barley
yeast)	Oats (cooked)	Buckwheat	Cereal (dry)	Oats (cooked)	Buckwheat
Buckwheat	Pancakes	Corn	Couscous	Pancakes	Cereal (cold,
Cereals (cold,	Quinoa	Millet	Crackers	Pasta**	dry, & puffed)
dry, puffed)	Rice (all kinds)	Muesli**	Durum flour	Rice (brown	Corn
Corn	Seitan (wheat	Oats (dry)	Granola	& white)	Couscous
Couscous	"meat")	Polenta**	Oat bran	Rice cakes**	Crackers
Crackers	Sprouted wheat	Quinoa	Oats (cooked)	Wheat	Durum flour*
Granola	bread (Essene)	Rice (brown)**	Pancakes		Granola
Millet	Wheat	Rye	Pasta		Millet
Muesli			Rice (basmati,		Muesli
Oat bran			white, & wild)		Oat bran
Oats (dry)			Rice cakes		Oats (dry)
Pasta**			Seitan (wheat		Polenta
Polenta**			"meat")		Quinoa*
Rice cakes**			Spelt		Rice (basmati
Rye			Sprouted wheat		& wild)*
Sago			bread (Essene)		Rye
Spelt			Tapioca		Seitan (wheat
Tapioca			Wheat		"meat")
Wheat bran			Wheat bran		Spelt*
					Sprouted
					wheat bread

		LEGUMES		*ok in moderation **ok rarely	

Aduki beans	Lentils (red)*	Miso	Aduki beans	Kidney beans	Aduki beans
Black beans	Mung beans	Soy sauce	Black beans	Miso	Black beans
Black-eyed	Mung dal	Soy sausages	Black-eyed	Soy beans	Black-eyed
peas	Soy cheese*	Tur dal	peas	Soy cheese	peas
Chickpeas	Soy milk*	Urad dal	Chickpeas	Soy flour	Chickpeas
Kidney beans	Soy sauce*		Kidney beans	Soy powder	Lentils (brown
Lentils (brown)	Soy sausages*		Lentils (brown	Soy sauce	& red)
Lima beans	Tofu*		& red)	Tofu (cold)	Lima beans
Miso**	Tur dal		Lima beans	Urad dal	Mung beans*
Peas (dried)	Urad dal		Mung beans		Mung dal*
Pinto beans			Mung dal		Peas (dried)
Soy beans			Peas (dried)		Pinto beans
Soy flour			Pinto beans		Soy milk
Soy powder			Soy beans		Soy sausages
Split peas			Soy cheese		Split peas
Tempeh			Soy flour*		Tempeh
White beans			Soy milk		Tofu (hot)*
			Soy powder*		Tur dal
			Split peas		White beans
			Tempeh		
			Tofu		

DAIRY				*ok in moderation **ok rarely	
VATA		PITTA		KAPHA	
No	Yes	No	Yes	No	Yes
Cow's milk (powdered) Goat's milk (powdered) Yogurt (plain, frozen, & fruit)	*Most dairy is good!* Cheese (hard) Butter Buttermilk Cheese (hard)* Cheese (soft) Cottage cheese Cow's milk Ghee Goat's cheese Goat's milk Ice cream* Sour cream* Yogurt (diluted & spiced)	Butter (salted) Buttermilk unsalted, & Sour cream Yogurt (plain, frozen, & fruit)	Butter (unsalted) Cheese (soft, (unsalted)** not aged) Cottage cheese Cow's milk Ghee Goat's milk Goat's cheese (soft & unsalted) Ice cream Yogurt (freshly made & diluted)*	Butter (salted) Butter cheese Cheese (soft & hard) Cow's milk Ice cream Sour cream Yogurt (plain, frozen, & fruit)	Buttermilk* Cottage (from skimmed goat's milk) Ghee* Goat's cheese (unsalted & not aged)* Goat's milk (skimmed) Yogurt (diluted)
ANIMAL FOODS				*ok in moderation **ok rarely	
Lamb Pork Rabbit Turkey (white) Venison	Beef Buffalo Chicken (dark) Chicken (white)* Duck Eggs Fish (freshwater & sea) Salmon Sardines Seafood Shrimp Tuna fish Turkey (dark)	Beef Chicken (dark) Duck Eggs (yolk) Fish (sea) Lamb Pork Salmon Sardines Seafood Tuna fish Turkey (dark)	Buffalo Chicken (white) Eggs (whites only) Fish (freshwater) Rabbit Shrimp* Turkey (white) Venison	Beef Buffalo Chicken (dark) Duck Fish (sea) Lamb Pork Salmon Sardines Seafood Tuna fish Turkey (dark)	Chicken (white) Eggs Fish (freshwater) Rabbit Shrimp Turkey (white) Venison

CONDIMENTS					*ok in moderation **ok rarely	
VATA		PITTA		KAPHA		
No	Yes	No	Yes	No	Yes	
Chocolate	Black pepper*	Chili peppers	Black pepper*	Chocolate	Black pepper	
Horseradish	Chili peppers*	Chocolate	Coriander	Gomasio	Chili peppers	
	Coriander	Gomasio	leaves	Kelp	Coriander	
	leaves*	Horseradish	Dulse*	Ketchup**	leaves	
	Dulse	Kelp	Hijiki*	Lime	Dulse*	
	Gomasio	Ketchup	Kombu*	Lime pickle	Hijiki*	
	Hijiki	Lemon	Lime*	Mango chutney	Horseradish	
	Kelp	Lime pickle	Mango chutney	(sweet)	Lemon*	
	Ketchup	Mango chutney	(sweet)	Mango pickle	Mango chutney	
	Lemon	(spicy)	Sprouts	Mayonnaise	(spicy)	
	Lime	Mango pickle	Tamari*	Pickles	Mustard	
	Lime pickle	Mayonnaise		Salt	(without	
	Mango chutney	Mustard		Soy sauce	vinegar)	
	(sweet & spicy)	Pickles		Tamari	Seaweed*	
	Mango pickle	Salt (in excess)		Vinegar	Spring onions	
	Mayonnaise	Seaweed			Sprouts	
	Mustard	Soy sauce				
	Pickles	Spring onions				
	Salt	Vinegar				
	Soy sauce					
	Spring onions					
	Sprouts*					
	Tamari					
	Vinegar					

NUTS					*ok in moderation **ok rarely	
None	In moderation:	Almonds	Almonds	Almonds	None	
	Almonds	(with skin)	(soaked	(soaked		
	Black walnuts	Black walnuts	& peeled)	& peeled)**		
	Brazil nuts	Brazil nuts	Coconuts	Black walnuts		
	Cashews	Cashews		Brazil nuts		
	Coconuts	Filberts		Cashews		
	Filberts	Hazelnuts		Coconuts		
	Hazelnuts	Macadamia		Filberts		
	Macadamia	nuts		Hazelnuts		
	nuts	Peanuts		Macadamia		
	Peanuts	Pecans		nuts		
	Pecans	Pine nuts		Peanuts		
	Pine nuts	Pistachios		Pecans		
	Pistachios	Walnuts		Pine nuts		
	Walnuts			Pistachios		
				Walnuts		

Appendix 1: Food Guidelines for Basic Constitutional Types

SEEDS				*ok in moderation **ok rarely	
VATA		**PITTA**		**KAPHA**	
No	Yes	No	Yes	No	Yes
Popcorn Psyllium**	Flax Halvah Pumpkin Sesame Sunflower Tahini	Sesame Tahini	Flax Halvah Popcorn (no salt, buttered) Psyllium Pumpkin*	Halvah Psyllium** Sesame Tahini	Flax* Popcorn (no salt, no butter) Pumpkin* Sunflower*

OILS				*ok in moderation **ok rarely	
Flax seed	*For internal & external use (most suitable at top of list):* Ghee Olive Sesame Most other oils *External use only:* Avocado Coconut	Almond Apricot Corn Safflower Sesame	*For internal & external use (most suitable at top of list):* Canola Flax seed Ghee Olive Primrose Soy Sunflower Walnut *External use only:* Avocado Coconut	Apricot Avocado Coconut Flax seed** Olive Safflower Sesame (internal) Soy Walnut	*For internal & external use in small amounts (most suitable at top of list):* Almond Canola Corn Ghee Sesame (external) Sunflower

BEVERAGES				*ok in moderation **ok rarely	
VATA		**PITTA**		**KAPHA**	
No	Yes	No	Yes	No	Yes
Apple juice	Alcohol (beer	Alcohol (spirits	Alcohol	Alcohol (beer,	Alcohol (dry
Black tea	& wine)*	& wine)	(beer)*	spirits &	wine, red
Caffeinated	Almond milk	Apple cider	Almond milk	sweet wine)	& white)
beverages	Aloe vera	Berry juice	Aloe vera juice	Almond milk	Aloe vera juice
Carbonated	juice	(sour)	Apple juice	Caffeinated	Apple cider
drinks	Apple cider	Caffeinated	Apricot juice	beverages**	Apple juice*
Chocolate	Apricot juice	beverages	Berry juice	Carbonated	Apricot juice
milk	Berry juice	Carbonated	(sweet)	drinks	Berry juice
Coffee	(except	drinks	Black tea*	Cherry juice	Black tea
Cold dairy	cranberry)	Carrot juice	Carob	(sour)	(spiced)
drinks	Carob*	Cherry juice	Chai *	Chocolate	Carob
Cranberry	Carrot juice	(sour)	Cherry juice	milk	Carrot juice
juice	Chai	Chocolate	(sweet)	Coffee	Chai*
Ice cold	Cherry juice	milk	Cool dairy	Cold dairy	Cherry juice
drinks	Grain "coffee"	Coffee	drinks	drinks	(sweet)
Iced tea	Grapefruit	Cranberry	Grain "coffee"	Grapefruit	Cranberry
Pear juice	juice	juice	Grape juice	juice	juice
Pomegranate	Grape juice	Grapefruit	Mango juice	Ice cold drinks	Grain "coffee"
juice	Lemonade	juice	Miso broth*	Iced tea	Grape juice
Prune juice**	Mango juice	Ice cold drinks	V-8 juice	Lemonade	Mango juice
Soy milk	Miso broth	Iced tea	Orange juice*	Miso broth	Peach nectar
(cold)	Orange juice	Lemonade	Peach nectar	Orange juice	Pear juice
Tomato juice**	Papaya juice	Papaya juice	Pear juice	Papaya juice	Pineapple
V-8 juice	Peach nectar	Pineapple	Pomegranate	Rice milk	juice*
	Pineapple	juice	juice	Sour juices	Pomegranate
	juice	Sour juices	Prune juice	Soy milk (cold)	juice
	Rice milk	Tomato juice	Rice milk	Tomatojuice	Soy milk (hot
	Sour juices	V-8 juice	Soy milk	V-8 juice	& well spiced)
	Soy milk (hot		Vegetable		
	& well-spiced)*		bouillon		
	Vegetable				
	bouillon				

BEVERAGES (continued)				*ok in moderation **ok rarely	
VATA		PITTA		KAPHA	
No	Yes	No	Yes	No	Yes
Herb teas:	*Herb teas:*	*Herb teas:*	*Herb teas:*	*Herb teas:*	*Herb teas:*
Alfalfa**	Ajwan	Ajwan	Alfalfa	Liquorice**	Alfafa
Barley**	Bancha	Basil**	Bancha	Marshmallow	Bancha
Basil**	Catnip*	Clove	Barley	Red Zinger	Barley
Blackberry	Chamomile	Eucalyptus	Blackberry	Rosehip**	Blackberry
Borage**	Chicory*	Fenugreek	Borage	Fenugreek	Burdock
Burdock	Chrysanthemum*	Ginger (dry)	Burdock		Chamomile
Cinnamon**	Clove	Ginseng	Catnip		Chicory
Cornsilk	Comfrey	Hawthorn	Chamomile		Cinnamon
Dandelion	Elderflower	Juniper berry	Chicory		Clove
Ginseng	Eucalyptus	Pennyroyal	Comfrey		Comfrey*
Hibiscus	Fennel	Red Zinger	Dandelion		Dandelion
Hops**	Fenugreek	Rosehip**	Fennel		Ginger
Jasmine**	Ginger (fresh)	Sage	Ginger (fresh)		Ginseng*
Lemon	Hawthorn	Sassafras	Hibiscus		Hibiscus
balm**	Juniper berry	Yerba maté	Hops		Jasmine
Nettle**	Kukicha*		Jasmine		Juniper berry
Passion	Lavender		Kukicha		Kukicha
flower**	Lemon grass		Lavender		Lavender
Red clover**	Licorice		Lemon balm		Lemon balm
Red Zinger**	Marshmallow		Lemon grass		Lemon grass
Violet**	Oat straw		Licorice		Nettle
Yarrow	Orange peel		Marshmallow		Passion
Yerba maté**	Pennyroyal		Nettle		flower
	Peppermint		Oat straw		Peppermint
			Passion		Raspberry
			flower		Red clover
					Sarsaparilla*
					Sassafras

SWEETENERS				*ok in moderation **ok rarely	
Maple syrup**	Barley malt	White sugar**	Barley malt	Barley malt	Fruit juice
White sugar	Fructose	Honey**	Fructose	Fructose	concentrates
	Fruit juice	Jaggery	Fruit juice	Jaggery	Honey (raw)
	concentrates	Molasses	concentrates	Maple syrup	
	Honey		Maple syrup	Molasses	
	Jaggery		Rice syrup	Rice syrup	
	Molasses		Turbinado	Turbinado	
	Rice syrup			White sugar	
	Turbinado				

SPICES *ok in moderation **ok rarely					
VATA		PITTA		KAPHA	
No	Yes	No	Yes	No	Yes
Caraway	All spices are good! Ajwan Allspice Almond extract Anise Asafetida (hing) Basil Bay leaves Black pepper Cardamom Cayenne* Cinnamon Cloves Coriander Cumin Dill Fennel Fenugreek* Garlic	Ajwan Allspice Almond extract Anise Asafetida (hing) Basil (dry) Bay leaves Cayenne Cloves Fenugreek Garlic Ginger (dry) Mace Marjoram Mustard seeds Nutmeg Oregano Paprika Pippali Poppy seeds Rosemary	Basil (fresh) Black pepper* Caraway* Cardamom* Cinnamon Coriander Cumin Dill Fennel Ginger (fresh) Mint Neem leaves* Orange peel* Parsley* Peppermint Saffron Spearmint Tarragon* Turmeric Vanilla* Wintergreen	Salt	All spices are good! Ajwan Allspice Almond extract Anise Asafetida (hing) Basil Bay leaves Black pepper Caraway Cardamom Cayenne Cinnamon Cloves Coriander Cumin Dill Fennel* Fenugreek
FOOD SUPPLEMENTS *ok in moderation **ok rarely					
Barley green Brewer's yeast	Aloe vera juice* Amino acids Bee pollen Blue-green algae Royal jelly Spirolina Vitamins A, B, B12, C, D, & E Minerals: Calcium Copper Iron Magnesium Zinc	Amino acids Bee pollen** Royal jelly** Vitamins A, B, B12 & C Minerals: Copper Iron	Aloe vera juice Barley green Blue-green algae Brewer's yeast Spirolina Vitamins D & E Minerals: Calcium Magnesium Zinc	Minerals: Potassium	Aloe vera juice Amino acids Barley green Bee pollen Blue-green algae Brewer's yeast Royal jelly Spirolina Vitamins A, B, B12, C, D, & E Minerals: Calcium Copper Iron Magnesium Zinc

Appendix 2

HERBAL REMEDIES

Triphala

"When in doubt, give *triphala*" could easily be the Ayurvedic motto. Triphala (the "three fruits") can be used to shampoo the hair or wash the body, as an emetic or a laxative, as nose, ear, or eye drops, as a gargle or a snuff, and as a decoction for enema. When eaten, it gently scrapes ama away from it, and also rejuvenates the membrane lining the digestive tract. It helps calm inflammations, scrapes excess fat from the body, and balances all three doshas. It is an ingredient in a large number of medicines and its three constituents are also made into a number of rejuvenating preparations.

Triphala is a mixture of *amalaki, haritaki,* and *bibhitaki.* Amalaki *(Emblica officinalis)* calms all three doshas, but pitta in particular. The *Charaka Samhita* says amalaki is the best of medicines for preventing aging. It is the main ingredient in the famous medicinal jam *chyavanaprasha,* which is used for treating respiratory complaints and for rejuvenation. Haritaki *(Terminalia chebula)* also calms all three doshas, but its main effect is on vata (prolonged use of haritaki alone, however, may aggravate vata). It scrapes ama away from the tissues, especially from the digestive tract, and rejuvenates the body, especially the colon and lungs. Bibhitaki *(Terminalia belerica)* again calms all three doshas, its main effect being on kapha. The unripe fruit is laxative, while the dried ripe fruit stops diarrhea, for which it is particularly effective. It also benefits hemorrhoids and skin diseases.

The combination of these three gives a result that is far greater than the sum of its parts. While triphala is not really specific for female complaints, the fact that it is unsurpassed in the realms of ridding the body of old amassed ama and regularizing the digestive tract makes it useful for almost any woman whose monthly cycle is distressed. Sometimes triphala on its own is enough to rearrange things, and even if it is not, it "gets the ball rolling" so that the next remedy will have less work to do.

Start with a half teaspoon of triphala at night just before bed. A good way to take it is to put it into boiling water, let it steep, and drink the result. But triphala is an acquired taste, and you may prefer simply to put the powder on your tongue and quickly wash it down with warm water. If you insist, you may put it into capsules or consume triphala tablets, but—as with food—the taste of medicine creates part of its effect, and it is good to experience at least a bit of its flavor as it goes down.

Sometimes an individual's body contains so much ama that when triphala mobilizes it, the ama tries to come out all at once, through the skin. This can sometimes produce a rash, which is not triphala's fault; it is the product of your own toxins. If this should happen to you, just stop taking the triphala until the rash goes away, then return to it in half the previous dose for a week or two until your body gets its elimination systems running properly.

You can take triphala for six months at a time, and if you have a preexisting condition it may be useful to take it for a year or more. Eventually, though, you will want to interrupt it for a few weeks or months, so that your system does not become habituated to it. You can always return to it later.

As a douche, triphala helps to scrape ama from the vagina and cervix. Boil one teaspoon in one pint of water for five to ten minutes, steep, and strain. Lie in the bath, insert the warm—not hot!—tea, and retain it as long as possible.

Aloe Vera

Aloe vera is one of the best tools we have to help regulate the monthly cycle. In Ayurveda, aloe is called *kumari* ("the maiden"), which suggests both that it contains the healthy energy of a young woman and that it tones the female organs. You can begin by taking one tablespoon of its juice or gel per day, mixed with pomegranate juice, some sweet juice (like grape or apple), or cooled hibiscus or fennel tea. Begin at the end of a period. Try to get a variety of aloe vera which is not preserved with either citric acid or ascorbic acid (even though ascorbic acid is vitamin C, it is still an acid, and acids increase pitta). If aloe agrees with you, increase the amount you take to 4 tablespoons twice a day, and continue for as long as needed (interrupting it during each menstrual period). If your stools become loose, you'll know you have taken too much.

Aloe is truly excellent for relieving excess menstrual flow and pain during menses, and for regularizing periods. You can also apply fresh aloe gel externally to burns, rashes, inflammations, insect bites, and other painful conditions. Aloe soothes and heals the whole body, but is particularly effective for relieving "acid" stomach, gastritis, and peptic ulcer, and for cooling pitta in the liver, blood, eyes, and digestion.

Shatavari

The root of *shatavari (Asparagus racemosus),* which is a relative of the vegetable asparagus, controls all three doshas, especially vata and pitta. It rejuvenates the blood and the female organs, helps to build up the body, strengthens the immune system, increases milk and sexual secretions, improves intellect, digestion, and physical strength, and strengthens the urinary tract. It can be used in any pitta condition in which ama is absent, for given in excess or to someone whose digestion is weak it may increase ama. Shatavari is usually consumed as a powder, a medicated ghee, or simmered in milk.

Ashvagandha

Ashvagandha (Withania somnifera) is a good tonic for a woman whose vata is high. It also helps to control kapha; in excess, it may increase pitta or ama. It is aphrodisiac and tonic and is mainly used to combat debility due to old age, nervous exhaustion, and simple overwork. It nurtures and clarifies the mind, calms and strengthens the nerves, and promotes sound, restful sleep. It rejuvenates and rebuilds body and mind, and relieves such conditions as rheumatism, consumption, infertility, emaciation, and weakness of the nerves. In small amounts it is a good tonic for weak pregnant women, but it must be used with care because large amounts have caused abortion.

Licorice

Licorice root *(Glycyrrhiza glabra)*—the herb, not the candy!— reduces vata and pitta, but increases kapha after long-term use by causing salt and water retention and loss of potassium. Licorice soothes sore throats and eases hoarseness, dilates the respiratory tract to ease breathing and promote expectoration of mucus (its effects are comparable to those of cortisone), reduces bleeding, and is aphrodisiac. One way to regulate a pitta- or vata-aggravated menstrual cycle is to drink one cup of licorice tea (steeped, not boiled) twice a day between periods. Licorice can act both as an emetic and a laxative; it improves the eyesight, strength, sexual power, and complexion, and strengthens the hair. It increases the production of reproductive juices and rejuvenates the system. Chewing on a licorice stem allays thirst, burning sensations, loss of appetite, cough, fatigue, and emaciation.

Musta

Known as nutgrass or knotgrass in the United States, where it is a rampant weed, *musta (Cyperus rotundus)* reduces pitta and kapha and regulates the menses. Even the ancient Romans used it as an emmenagogue, a substance that promotes the menstrual flow. It digests ama without aggravating pitta. As a weak decoction in water it is given for fevers, diarrhea, dysentery, indigestion, and hemorrhoids. Its powder shows some fat-reducing activity.

Vetivert

Vetivert *(Vetiveria zizanyoides)* strongly reduces pitta, and also reduces kapha. Its root relieves thirst and burning sensations, and purifies and invigorates the blood, skin, and genitourinary tract. It strengthens the digestive fire, digests ama, and calms both vomiting and diarrhea. It purifies sweat and urine; a strong decoction, cooled, is good for inflammation of the urinary tract or the reproductive organs, and a weak decoction, cooled, can be sipped during high fevers. It benefits almost all pitta-caused inflammations, and its paste makes a good cooling application for pitta-induced skin diseases or in "hot" fevers. Incense or essential oil of vetivert cools the mind and can improve concentration.

Brahmi

Known as *gotu kola* in the West, *brahmi (Centella asiatica,* syn. *Hydrocotyle asiatica)* balances all three doshas and stimulates the circulatory system, especially the blood vessels of the skin and the mucous membranes. It is a rejuvenative; it revitalizes the nerves and brain, strengthens memory and intelligence, promotes longevity, and improves concentration, voice, physical strength, digestive power, and complexion. Brahmi controls pitta and has been used in pitta-caused fevers, skin diseases, and afflictions of the reproductive organs. It is often taken internally as a medicated ghee, otherwise as a tea or extract. Oil medicated with brahmi is used to promote hair growth and to "refrigerate" the brain.

Guggulu

Guggulu is the resin of a small tree *(Commiphora mukul)*. It controls and balances all three doshas, although theoretically, excessive use might increase pitta. It stimulates the skin, mucous membranes, and kidneys to excrete toxins, it scrapes ama and fat from the tissues, purifies the blood, strengthens the nerves, and rejuvenates the body. It reduces blood cholesterol, increases white blood cells, and stimulates phagocytosis (the process by which the white cells engulf and devour alien invaders in the body). Guggulu relieves pain, strengthens the thyroid, and raises the blood level of thyroid hormone; it may counteract the action of melatonin. Its strong anti-inflammatory action makes guggulu the best medicine for many kinds of arthritis. It also helps relieve vaginal discharges, although its cousin *myrrh (Commiphora myrrha)* may be even more effective at purifying and rejuvenating the female reproductive tract. It is an emmenagogue (a substance which promotes the menstrual flow) and analgesic, and seems to show some antifertility activity. Guggulu has been used successfully in India to treat such diseases as hepatitis and myocardial necrosis (destruction of heart tissue after a heart attack).

Guggulu is an excellent *yogavahi* (a compound which carries the other substances mixed with it deep into the tissues); when added to a compound, it potentiates its fellow ingredients. It is therefore usually used in combination. *Yogaraja guggulu,* which contains almost three dozen herbs, is given in rheumatism and rheumatoid arthritis, gout, diseases of the nerves, hemorrhoids, epilepsy, urinary diseases, heart disease, anemia, and other conditions in which vata is aggravated. Despite guggulu's antifertility activity, yogaraja guggulu is said to improve the fertility of both men and women, probably by removing ama that is impeding it. *Kaishora guggulu* contains *guduchi (Tinospora cordifolia),* which has been shown to be an immunomodulator. Although guduchi cures all three doshas, it is mainly used for pitta problems, and there are few pitta-caused conditions it cannot tackle. It can also be used as powder or *sattva* (starchy water extract).

The guggulu formula most used to reduce excess body fat is *triphala guggulu*, which should be taken twice a day after a meal (one or two pills at a time is enough!), with warm water or a tea of dry ginger. Although the triphala that it contains will purify your system as it scrapes away fat, like all other Ayurvedic preparations triphala guggulu works better once you have already begun to purify your system. One way to do this is to use castor oil before you start triphala guggulu. If you are at least forty pounds heavier than your ideal weight, or your cholesterol is significantly higher than normal, you may wish to facilitate triphala guggulu's scraping action by taking castor oil each morning for six weeks, washing it down with a cup of tea of dry ginger. Begin with one teaspoon of castor oil, and try to work your way up to one tablespoon (it should not produce a laxative effect). After six weeks, your system will be ready for triphala guggulu.

If you want to use one of the guggulu compounds for countering rheumatoid arthritis or some similar disorder that requires an anti-inflammatory effect, you might begin with a more intensive castor oil cleansing. After bathing or showering one morning, take four teaspoons of castor oil and wash it down with one or more cups of tea of dry ginger (not too strong), which you have sweetened slightly with jaggery or molasses. Keep sipping this tea over the next few hours, during which time you will probably experience two to four bowel movements. Once your intestines appear to have emptied themselves fully and calmed down, have a light meal of mung bean soup and rice or mung bean khichadi (see page 80), and go to bed early. Keep your diet simple over the next few days as your digestive fire regains its strength. This type of castor oil "purge" can also be a useful way to "re-ignite" your digestion when it seems totally out of whack, even in the absence of a chronic condition—but don't overdo it.

Chandra Prabha and Shilajit

Chandra prabha is a wonderful pill made of a number of herbs (including triphala) plus iron, guggulu, and *shilajit*, a tarry substance that purifies and strengthens the genitals and the urinary tract. A many-talented pill, chandra prabha can help to relieve kapha-caused vaginal discharges and ovarian cysts, and when given with shatavari and aloe vera it can regulate most irregular cycles. It also has an ama-reducing and fat-scraping effect, and reduces blood sugar. However, it must be used with care in pitta conditions. The Ayurvedically prepared iron *(loha bhasma)* in chandra prabha facilitates the scraping of ama and other wastes from the system, and it also helps to replace iron that is lost in the flow.

Shilajit is sometimes used in other combinations for diabetes, edema, and reproductive and urinary disorders. It is a powerful aphrodisiac and stimulant, and is given as a rejuvenator in consumption, chronic bronchitis, asthma, chronic digestive diseases, nervous conditions, and the like.

Other Remedies

Bala means "strength," and bala root (*Sida* species) is sweet, aphrodisiac, rejuvenative, unctuous, and cooling. It strengthens the tissues and the nervous system. Bermuda grass, a reviled weed in the United States, controls all three doshas and cures diseases due to pitta and kapha. While it dries excessive fluids, especially lymph, blood, fat, and urine, its main use is to stop bleeding. The fresh juice is instilled in the nose for nosebleeds, used as enemas for bleeding hemorrhoids, or colitis, and is taken internally—as much as one ounce of juice every fifteen minutes—to relieve excessive menstrual flow.

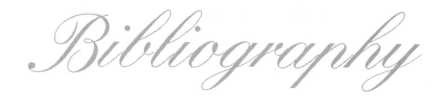

Bibliography

Diamond, Dr. Jared. "Sex and the Female Agenda." *Discover,* September 1993.

———. "Why Women Change." *Discover,* July 1996.

Dossey, M.D., Larry. *Healing Words.* New York: HarperCollins, 1993.

Kingsolver, Barbara. *Pigs in Heaven.* New York: HarperCollins, 1993.

Lad, Usha, and Dr. Vasant Lad. *Ayurvedic Cooking for Self-Healing.* Albuquerque: The Ayurvedic Press, 1994.

Lad, Dr. Vasant. *Ayurveda: The Science of Self-Healing,* (second edition). Santa Fe: Lotus Press, 1985.

———. *The Complete Book of Ayurvedic Home Remedies.* Nevada City, Nev.: Harmony Books, 1998.

———. *Secrets of the Pulse: The Ancient Art of Ayurvedic Pulse Diagnosis.* Albuquerque: The Ayurvedic Press, 1996.

Lad, Dr. Vasant, and David Frawley. *The Yoga of Herbs: An Ayurvedic Guide to Herbal Medicine.* Santa Fe: Lotus Press, 1986.

Lonsdorf, M.D., Nancy, Veronica Butler, M.D., and Melanie Brown, Ph.D. *A Woman's Best Medicine: Health, Happiness, and Long Life Through Maharishi Ayur-Veda.* New York: Jeremy P. Tarcher/Putnam,1995.

Mehta, P. M., ed. *Charaka Samhita.* Jamnagar: Gulab Kunverba Society, 1949.

Morningstar, Amadea. *The Ayurvedic Cookbook*. Santa Fe: Lotus Press, 1986.

Northrup, Christiane. *Women's Bodies, Women's Wisdom*. New York: Bantam Books, 1994.

Srikantamurthy, K. R., trans. *Ashtanga Hrdayam*. Varanasi: Krishnadas Academy, 1991.

Srikantamurthy, K. R., trans. *Sharngadhara Samhita*. Varanasi: Chaukhambha Orientalia, 1984.

Svoboda, Robert E. *Ayurveda: Life, Health and Longevity*. London: Penguin, 1992.

———. *The Greatness of Saturn*. Floresville, Tex.: Sadhana Publications, 1997.

———. *The Hidden Secret of Ayurveda*. Albuquerque: The Ayurvedic Press, 1994.

———. *Prakruti: Your Ayurvedic Constitution*. Albuquerque: Geocom, 1988.

———. *Tao and Dharma*. Sante Fe: Lotus Press, 1995.

Tisdale, Sallie. *Talk Dirty to Me*. New York: Doubleday, 1994.

Van Howten, Donald. *Ayurveda and Life Impressions Bodywork— Seeking Our Healing Memories*. Sante Fe: Lotus Press, 1997.

Resources

The Ayurvedic Institute
P.O. Box 23445
Albuquerque, NM 87192-1445
Telephone: 505-291-9698; Fax: 505-294-7572

Directed by Dr. Vasant Lad, the Institute includes a school providing in-depth teaching of Ayurveda, an herb department, private consultations and panchakarma, and a correspondence course written by Dr. Robert Svoboda on the basics of Ayurveda. Dr. Svoboda's *Ayurvedic Home Study Course* can be ordered from this address.

EthnicSuperStore.com
Website: www.EthnicSuperStore.com

This online grocery store offers a comprehensive selection of Indian foods and spices.

Sushakti
1840 Iron St., Suite C
Bellingham, WA 98225
Telephone: 360-752-0575; Fax: 360-752-9831
E-mail: info@ayurveda-sushakti.com
Website: www.ayurveda-sushakti.com

This company offers Ayurvedic books, herbs, and a range of skincare products.

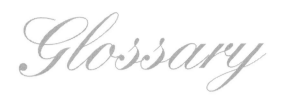

Glossary

Agni: Literally, fire, in all its aspects. Agni encompasses all fires, from the densest (the power of digestion) to the most rarefied (the essence of cosmic fire).

Ama: A general term for internal toxins produced by improper metabolic functioning, especially toxins that result from the mis-digestion of food and from "mis-digested" mental and emotional experiences.

Apana vata: The downward-moving air, one of vata's five subdoshas, which divide the body into five spheres of influence. Apana is responsible for expelling things from the body.

Artava: Broadly, female reproductive tissue and "juices," and the metabolic processes involved in their formation.

Ashtanga Hridraya of Vagbhata: The Ayurvedic text used most widely today, written about 700 A.D., formed by condensing *Charaka Samhita* and *Sushruta Samhita* and including newly described diseases and therapies.

Charaka Samhita: One of the first substantial texts on Ayurveda, first compiled about 3,000 years ago and dealing mainly with internal medicine.

Dhara: An Ayurvedic treatment in which a liquid, often oil, is continuously poured on the forehead for a half-hour to an hour and a half.

Dosha: Literally, fault, mistake, imperfection. There are three doshas—see vata, pitta, and kapha. Doshas are invisible forces that cannot be perceived directly, but are responsible for all biological and psychological functions in the mind and body. The three doshas pervade the body, working in every cell at every instant. Their actions can be demonstrated through the bodily substances that are their vehicles. The doshas preserve an organism's balance and rhythm when they are themselves balanced, and disturb the organism's harmony when they are disturbed. Each dosha has five varieties, or subdoshas.

Ghee: Clarified butter, prepared by simmering unsalted butter on the lowest possible heat until all the water boils off and then straining out the milk solids. The purified fat remaining is the ghee, which is easier to digest than butter. When properly digested, ghee promotes production of ojas.

Jyotish: Indian systems of astrology.

Kapha: One of the three doshas, comprising the water and earth elements (see mahabhutas). The principle of potential energy that stabilizes an organism.

Khichadi: A dish prepared from split legumes (usually mung beans) and rice.

Mahabhutas: The five great elements, or five great states of material existence: space (ether), air, fire, water, and earth.

Ojas: The subtle glue that integrates body, mind, and spirit together into a functioning individual. A hormone-like substance, it is derived from *shukra* and *artava*. Ojas produces the aura, it transmits energy from mind to body, and controls immunity.

Panchakarma: Active purification methods, including emesis (vomiting), purgation, medicated enema, nasal medications, and blood-letting. These should only be carried out under the guidance of a trained practitioner and after proper preparation of the body.

Pitta: One of the three doshas, comprising the fire and water elements (see mahabhutas). The force in charge of all transformation in the organism and controlling the balance of its kinetic and potential energies.

Pizhichil: Specialized Ayurvedic oil application, whereby heated medicated oil is applied to the limbs.

Prajnaparadha: Literally, an offense against wisdom. A perversity of mind that acts willfully in a way known to be unhealthy or detrimental to your well-being.

Prakriti: Literally, first action. An individual's inherent nature or constitution, the inborn tendencies that influence consciousness and activity. Prakriti determines which response your body or mind first displays to a stress.

Prana: The life force.

Prana vata: The forward-moving air, one of vata's five subdoshas, which divide the body into five spheres of influence. Prana regulates what comes into the system.

Rasa: A word with many meanings depending on context, but encompassing everything that is "juicy" in one's existence, including tastes (especially the six tastes of Ayurveda) and the emotions derived from them; lymph and blood plasma, semen, and milk.

Rasayana: Rejuvenation practices to return your body-mind-spirit complex to an earlier state of natural integration, to prevent diseases that are preventable, and to minimize those that cannot be avoided.

Rishis: Seers, enlightened experimenters who worked within the "laboratories" of their own awareness to "perceive" the fundamentals of Ayurveda.

Ritam: Divinely permanent and invincible order, the source of all our more limited and temporary human harmonies.

Samana vata: The equalizing air, one of vata's five subdoshas, which divide the body into five spheres of influence. Samana supervises digestion and assimilation.

Shakti: Energy or power, including the power of creation.

Shukra: Broadly, male reproductive tissue and "juices" and the metabolic processes involved in their formation.

Sushruta Samhita: One of the first substantial texts on Ayurveda, first compiled about 3,000 years ago and dealing with surgery.

Svastha: Literally, to be established in yourself. Healthy.

Svastha vritta: Literally, establishing oneself in good habits. Preventive medicine.

Tejas: The essence of cosmic fire, which controls the mind's digestion and is transmitted via ojas into the body's digestive system.

Udana vata: The upward-moving air, one of vata's five subdoshas that divide the body into five spheres of influence. Udana controls self-expression.

Vajikarana: Virilization, which is rejuvenation for your reproductive organs and "pre-juvenation" for your children—a way to select healthy genes with which to create a child with a healthy constitution.

Vanaprastha: Literally, forest-dwelling. A reflective phase in the post-menopausal years in which to digest your life's experiences, allowing a layer of wisdom—which deepens and enriches the flavor of your life's sweetness—gradually to rise to the top of your churning awareness.

Vata: One of the three doshas, comprising the air and space (ether) elements (see **mahabhutas**). The body's principle of kinetic energy, in charge of all motion in the body and mind.

Vedas: India's ancient books of wisdom.

Vikriti: The changeable current state of a person's health, which is a temporary condition expressed as the current state of the three doshas and can be different from the constitutional balance of the doshas, or **prakriti**.

Vrata: Vows, an ancient Vedic spiritual tradition of women.

Vrata katha: Vow stories, told to pass cultural and spiritual knowledge from generation to generation.

Vyadhikshamatva: Literally, forgiveness of disease. Immunity.

Vyana vata: The pervasive air, one of vata's five subdoshas that divide the body into five spheres of influence. Vyana is responsible for circulation and the distribution of nourishment.

Index

life-extension, 52–53, 141, 160
life-force. *See* prana

Macaulay, Lord, 2
mace, 104–5, 155
mangoes, 81, 147
marriage/singlehood, 113–15.
    See also relationships
massage
    for adolescents, 52
    dhara, 140
    and exercise, 63
    for infants, 38–40
    and the menstrual cycle, 77
    pizhichil, 140
    in postmenopausal years, 140
    during pregnancy, 121
    and purification regimens, 30, 31
    and skin care, 89
meats, 81, 90, 96, 150
meditation, 30, 53, 57–59, 63, 76
melatonin, 161
melons, 97, 147
memory, 102, 160
men
    distinctions of, 109–10
    hormones in, 29, 110–11
    and marriage, 113–15
    oppression of women by, 112–13
    and orgasm, 107–8
    and premature ejaculation, 105
    and relationships, 117–18
    and sexual communion, 115–17
menopause, 30. *See also* osteoporosis;
    womanhood, postmenopause
    attitudes about, 135–36
    and diet, 137–38
    and hormone replacement, 139, 141

and illness, 140
purpose of, 134–35
symptoms of, 135, 136–37
and vata, 136
Menstrual Channel, 6–7
menstrual cycle, 29, 70–71.
    See also menopause; monthly
    dysfunction syndrome;
    premenstrual syndrome
and ama, 71
amenorrhea, 48, 74, 102
and breathing, 79
and creativity, 6–7, 31, 45–46
and diet, 75, 79–83
and the doshas, 29, 45, 71,
    73–75
and hormones, 110
menarche, 30, 44–46
menstrual hut, 72
and purification regimens, 77–78
seasons of, 30
and sexuality, 108
mentors, 56–57, 132, 142
metabolic disorders, 55
migraine. *See* headaches
Milk Channel, 6–7
milk, warm, 106, 121
mind-body medicine, 9
mineral supplements, 50–51, 137,
    138, 155, 163
monogamy, 111–12. *See also*
    marriage; relationships
monthly dysfunction syndrome,
    72–73. *See also* premenstrual
    syndrome (PMS)
causes of, 75–76
and kapha, 74–75
and pitta, 74, 76